# NEW YORK AFTER 9/11

# NEW YORK AFTER 9/11

## SUSAN OPOTOW AND ZACHARY BARON SHEMTOB,
### EDITORS

**Empire State Editions**
An imprint of Fordham University Press
New York 2018

Fordham University Press has no responsibility for the persistence or accuracy
of URLs for external or third-party Internet websites referred to in this
publication and does not guarantee that any content on such websites is, or will
remain, accurate or appropriate.

Fordham University Press also publishes its books in a variety of electronic
formats. Some content that appears in print may not be available in electronic
books.

Visit us online:
www.empirestateeditions.com
www.fordhampress.com

Library of Congress Cataloging-in-Publication Data available online at https://
catalog.loc.gov.

Printed in the United States of America

20 19 18     5 4 3 2 1

First edition

# Contents

# NEW YORK AFTER 9/11

# Introduction

Susan Opotow and Zachary Baron Shemtob

An estimated two billion people around the world watched the destruction of the World Trade Center in 2001. Everyone understood that a momentous event was occurring before their eyes, but what happened in the days, months, and years afterward is far less clear. At this time, when memory is becoming history, it is important to understand the long-term experience and influence of September 11 on New York.

*New York After 9/11* looks back on the aftermath of the terrorist attacks of September 11, 2001 from multiple vantage points. In chapters by experts in architecture, medicine, health, community advocacy, psychology, public safety, human rights, and law, the complex post–9/11 period unfolds. The authors describe issues, challenges, conflicts, cooperation, and successes and discuss details about well-known and lesser-known issues. Their valuable accounts explain firsthand experiences. Together, their chapters elucidate how a major city responded to a catastrophic and traumatic attack, the tumultuous and subtle changes that occurred in its wake, and key lessons from this period for the future.

Many recall the initial period after 9/11 as one of collective shock followed by a deep sense of cooperation and solidarity. There is less agreement about what happened next. When did this initial sense of unity splinter? Did the disagreements that followed—about designing sites of memory, policing communities, and balancing freedom and safety—make the city a worse or better place? How should we understand initiatives that proved catastrophically wrong, such as the decision to surveil Muslims? By grounding their chapters in concrete problems that emerged and actions taken in response to them, the authors present an authoritative and informative guide to what happened in wake of a catastrophic attack and the consequences of the resulting decisions. Their analyses allow us to understand how the events of September 11 and its immediate aftermath rippled out over time to affect New York City in the years since and into the present.

This book is written for people who care about cities and their resilience and who want to know more about the recent history of New York. As we will discuss, it is also a book for scholars and practitioners interested in disaster preparedness.

## September 11, 2001

On the morning of September 11, 2001, nineteen Al Qaeda–affiliated hijackers seized four commercial flights. Two of these flights, both Boeing 767 jets, flew into the North and South Towers of the World Trade Center within minutes of each other. Within two hours, both Towers collapsed. Of the 3,000 fatalities resulting from the attacks in New York City, Washington, and Shanksville, Pennsylvania, most (93 percent) occurred in Lower Manhattan. There, 157 people died aboard the two hijacked airplanes; 2,606 workers and visitors in the Towers lost their lives; and 343 firefighters, 60 police officers, and eight EMTs and paramedics died in rescue operations.[1]

In addition, the rapid collapse and disintegration of two very large structures, each 110 floors, produced a roiling cloud of toxic dust containing cement, gypsum, asbestos, glass fibers, calcium carbonate, lead, and other metal particles. In the months and years since, many people have become ill or died from exposure to toxins during rescue, cleanup, and recovery efforts, and many more have continued to experience physical and psychological aftereffects. As of September 2017, more than 80,000 people qualified for and were enrolled in the World Trade Center Health Program.

## Immediate Aftershocks

New York City—both people and the place—was grievously wounded by the scale and violence of death and destruction on 9/11. The shocking specter of people covered in white ash, ubiquitous police barricades, the persistent smell of smoke, and the many missing person signs throughout the city signaled that the city had been devastated and irrevocably changed.[2] At first, the attack disrupted routine patterns of life, shattered a sense of security, aroused fear of further attacks, and deeply distressed people in New York.[3] In the prolonged state of mourning and calamity that ensued, people, organizations, and governmental agencies responded as best they could. A spontaneous outpouring of grassroots initiatives included makeshift memorials throughout the city, notably in Union Square, and such creative projects as Here Is New York and the Sonic Memorial Project projects provided occasions for people to connect. These timely initiatives also contributed valuable historical visual, narrative, and sonic archives about September 11.[4]

The World Trade Center's destruction had significant financial repercussions as well.[5] It shut down one of the world's busiest commercial centers for weeks and destroyed property valued at billions of dollars. This resulted in an estimated $3 billion loss for New York City in the first two years after 9/11,[6] precipitating massive layoffs in 2001 and 2002 that affected 145,844 workers in 34 states.[7] The disaster had particularly adverse effects on low-wage workers such as taxi drivers and Chinatown garment workers.[8]

Plans for reconstruction that emerged shortly after the initial shock of the attack precipitated fears about a changing New York City.[9] Would redevelopment of the World Trade Center site change lower Manhattan and the city as a whole? Would New York City retain its identity as a melting pot? Would the voices of all—not just the economically and politically powerful—be heard as building plans proceeded?

In the weeks, months, and years that followed, the redevelopment of the World Trade Center site became increasingly prominent in the news as business, government, and community stakeholders with markedly different visions and priorities for the site clashed.[10] Lower Manhattan workers and residents formed groups to press public officials to respond to an emerging health crisis resulting from exposure to toxic matter.[11] Though city and federal agencies initially rebuffed their pleas, they ultimately acknowledged the legitimacy and seriousness of the concerns.[12]

Now that much time has passed, the authors of this book believe that an analysis of 9/11's aftermath is vital to document the many shifts, both obvious and subtle, that have taken place. *New York After 9/11* fills this need with chapters that analyze the post–9/11 period in key spheres of New York City life. It is intended to deepen readers' sense of the complexity and drama of post-disaster changes and how those changes have rippled into present-day life.

For interested readers, there is much to be learned from the detail in these accounts of challenges, conflicts, transitions, and accomplishments in September 11's aftermath. For policymakers, the book's analyses of post-disaster challenges in a large urban center offer a rich and informative resource for disaster preparedness. For researchers, the chapters offer important data on New York City's post-disaster trajectory over time.

Because September 11 was an unprecedented event that focused attention on Lower Manhattan, first as a site of trauma and then as a site of recovery, the next section attends to its history. We then describe each chapter's contribution to an understanding of the post–9/11 trajectory.

## Lower Manhattan's Historic Neighborhoods and Burial Ground

The World Trade Center complex, destroyed on September 11, 2001, consisted of seven buildings that opened on April 4, 1973. Its landmark Twin Towers were briefly the tallest buildings in the world. This project was conceived and spearheaded by banker David Rockefeller, who founded the Downtown–Lower Manhattan Association in 1958 to develop Lower Manhattan as a business center. Construction on the World Trade Center began in the 1960s on a site that had been a lively retail and warehouse district known as "Radio Row," dubbed a "tinkerer's paradise."[13] It had emerged as a neighborhood in 1921 with several city blocks occupied by small electronics stores that sold used radios, war surplus electronics, and other electronic equipment that was piled high in bins and on the sidewalks.

Little Syria, an earlier neighborhood, had occupied an area just south of the current World Trade Center site. Populated by immigrants from Ottoman-controlled Greater Syria (now Syria, Lebanon, Palestine, Israel, and Jordan), this neighborhood thrived from 1880 until the Immigration Act of 1924 closed off further migration to the United States. In the 1940s, Little Syria was demolished to make way for the Brooklyn-Battery Tunnel.[14] Few traces of it now remain, with the exception of the Downtown Community House and St. George Chapel.[15]

Five Points, a nineteenth-century neighborhood northeast of the current World Trade Center, now stereotyped as notorious because of gangs and crime, was a poor, working-class, and racially and ethnically diverse enclave with a lively popular culture.[16] The Five Points neighborhood thrived for seventy years but ceased to exist by the late 1800s when the city expanded and enveloped it. Major federal, state, and city buildings occupy much of it now.

Adjacent to Five Points is the African Burial Ground, the oldest and largest burial site for Africans and Black Americans in North America. It was discovered in 1991 when construction for a federal office building revealed skeletal remains. The burial ground contains remains of an estimated 15,000 African American people, both free and enslaved. The site offers valuable historic information about slavery's role in building New York City. It is now estimated that people with African ancestry comprised a quarter of New York's population at the time of the Revolutionary War.[17] In 1993 the burial ground was designated as a National Historic Landmark, and it became a National Monument in 2006.

Historical artifacts and documents from the African Burial Ground, 850,000 nineteenth-century historical objects from Five Points, and other important historical collections that had been stored in the Twin Towers were lost on 9/11 when the Towers were destroyed. Miraculously, some materials from the African Burial Ground were later recovered in the debris left by the Towers' collapse.[18]

*Lower Manhattan's Expanding Contours*

Daniel Libeskind observes that Lower Manhattan is an ancient site.[19] Its oldest artifact may be a forty-foot glacial pothole that had been carved in rock twenty thousand years before it was discovered during excavation at the World Trade Center's site after 2001.[20] Excavations in 2010 uncovered an eighteenth-century ship with wood dating to 1773.[21]

Well before Dutch settlers arrived in Manhattan in the seventeenth century, Munsee Lenape people lived in Lower Manhattan, an island they called Manahatta, "hilly island."[22] Manahatta's original Hudson River shoreline would bisect the World Trade Center site today. Lower Manhattan has been widening over the past four centuries due to human intervention. Dutch settlers dumped their refuse into the island's coves, wetlands, and bays, moving the Hudson River shoreline westward. Advancing this process in the eighteenth century, New York City sold "water lots" to entrepreneurs to encourage the use of landfill to create more buildable space. By 1847, Lower Manhattan was wider than it had been a century before, and by 1976, it widened even further when Battery Park City was created from earth and rock excavated from the World Trade Center's foundation.[23]

In 2012, Hurricane Sandy overwhelmed Lower Manhattan, flooding subway tunnels, setting back completion of the September 11 Memorial Museum,[24] and causing an estimated $33 billion in damages. Because the areas flooded were those that rested on four hundred years of accumulated landfill, the hurricane essentially retraced Manahatta's pre–seventeenth century contours.[25]

This brief history reveals parallels between the past and contemporary social issues, including the displacement and erasure of small business and low-income neighborhoods and the damaging effect of restrictive immigration laws on thriving communities. Few traces of Lower Manhattan's predecessor communities remain. The communities of Munsee Lenape people, African American residents of Manhattan, and the poor and working-class neighborhoods contrast sharply with the striking commercial, residential, cultural architecture and development rapidly altering Lower Manhattan today.

## Challenge, Conflict, and Change after September 11

Each of the chapters in *New York After 9/11* begins at time zero—September 11, 2001—and trace its sequelae, speaking to memory, health and safety, and conflict in specific contexts of city life. They describe, for example, rethinking public safety, physical and mental health, reconstruction of the World Trade Center site, and designing commemorative spaces. Because precedents for such a devastating attack were lacking, some policies instituted after 9/11 were shortsighted and harmful. The surveillance of Muslim Americans, for example, was a violation of rights and left a pernicious legacy in New York.[26] The failure to designate Ground Zero as a toxic site unnecessarily exposed rescuers, workers, residents, and school children to environmental contaminants.[27] Poor communication and power struggles among city and federal agencies charged with public safety conflicted with the best interests of the people in New York City.[28] And some decisions pitted the health and safety of communities and workers against the political and economic sectors, the latter of which wanted to get the city up and running as quickly as possible.[29] Chapters on the World Trade Center's master plan, building the September 11 Memorial, and the development of the September 11 Memorial Museum describe these many design, technical, political, fiscal, and emotional challenges involved in their development, as well as the significant contribution these initiatives made to recovery and urban life.

In the extended period after September 11, intergroup collaborations proved to be a vital resource. Throughout the book, there are many examples of this on a small and local as well as on the national scale, such as the advocacy by New York's congressional delegation to the US Congress to obtain federal funding to monitor and treat post–9/11 illness. Analyses of the successes and challenges that emerged in the extended aftermath of September 11 also offer an empirical resource for future disaster preparedness and policies. Overall, the chapters suggest that cooperation, transparency in decision making, and the inclusion of affected communities are vital in garnering the knowledge necessary to solve problems, issues, and conflicts that arise in the extended and complex period of recovery.

The book begins with "Conflict and Change: New York City's Rebirth after 9/11," in which Zachary Baron Shemtob, Patrick Sweeney, and Susan Opotow trace 9/11's impact on people most directly affected by the World Trade Center's destruction: the residents of New York City and Lower Manhattan. Using *New York Times* articles as data, the authors focus on New Yorkers' experiences of 9/11 in the first five years after this catastrophic event and then they examine the subsequent controversy in 2010 surrounding the so-called Ground Zero Mosque. Tracing the post–9/11 trajectory in both periods, the authors found that both periods involved debate about how to properly commemorate, respect, and move on; a clash between socioemotional and economic values; the waxing and eventual waning of the public voice; and questions of power and control. The authors conclude that the longer aftermath of a disaster is a multifaceted event, and they identify common priorities that emerge at both the individual and group levels.

In "Mirror Reflections: (Re)Constructing Memory and Identity in Hiroshima and New York City," Hirofumi Minami and Brian Davis compare posttrauma reconstructions of Ground Zero in two cities, Hiroshima and New York. Using a psychoanalytic framework, the authors observe that people in both cities had been reluctant to confront an historical memory that was experienced as unspeakable. They describe the importance of forging a collective memory that can "re-present" the past in light of the needs of the present, recognizing memories connected to Ground Zero while being attentive to a city's sense of its own identity. Ultimately, the authors argue that giving voice to deep layers of collective trauma can be liberating and foster a better future.

In "Memory Foundations," Daniel Libeskind describes the intent, challenges, and realization of his master plan for the redevelopment of the World Trade Center site. Libeskind sought to transform a tragic site into civic space for the people of New York. He did so by creating a design that was attentive to the balance between public space and commercial requirements, as well as to memory of the past and looking toward the future. The chapter discusses his plan from its inception to the present, as the new World Trade Center—still a work in progress —is revitalizing urban life in Lower Manhattan and New York City.

In "Building the 9/11 Memorial," Michael Arad describes his design for the National September 11 Memorial, *Reflecting Absence*, located on the plaza of the World Trade Center in Lower Manhattan. He discusses how his personal reaction to the 9/11 attacks influenced his design, which sought to make the memorial a living part of New York City while cognizant of the site's profound sadness. Arad describes challenges that have shaped the memorial's design and symbolic features and discusses how the National September 11 Memorial site has increasingly become part of New York City's fabric since its inauguration in September 2011.

In "Urban Security in NYC Post–9/11: Risks and Realities," Charles Jennings describes the challenges New York City's public safety agencies faced and the new duties they took on after 9/11. The post–9/11 influx of federal funds and the aggressive embrace of counterterrorism by the New York Police Department (NYPD), he notes, strengthened NYPD's power relative to its partner agencies, fire and emergency management. New York City's elected officials stepped back and did not exercise oversight as the NYPD undertook an expanded role in counterterrorism and continued its crime reduction strategies, leading to overreach on both fronts. He also discusses the media's role, both as a communicator of risk information to the public and as a tool for local officials to publicize their public safety efforts. Ultimately, Jennings proposes that New York City adopt more risk-informed patterns of communication in the future.

In "Managing Fire Emergencies in Tall Buildings: Design Innovations in the Wake of 9/11," Norman Groner examines technological and regulatory innovations following 9/11 that have improved safety in tall buildings. An important innovation is the use of specially designed elevators that can evacuate tall buildings efficiently and safely even during fire emergencies. He catalogues uneven trends in efforts to improve occupant safety in high-rise buildings since 9/11, and notes that safety risks cannot be completely eliminated. However, buildings in the United States and Europe are safer now than before, he observes, making it more likely that building occupants will survive routine emergencies as well as terrorist attacks.

In "Health Impacts of 9/11," Michael Crane, Kimberly Flynn, Roberto Lucchini, Guille Mejia, Jacqueline Moline, Micki Siegel de Hernandez, David Prezant, and Joan Reibman describe health issues that arose after 9/11 and the medical, logistical, political, and policy challenges they faced to get 9/11-related health conditions recognized and addressed. These authors are medical personnel from World Trade Center Health Program sites, labor union representatives, and Lower Manhattan community members who have worked together on post–September 11 health issues. Initially, their efforts to get emerging health problems related to the disaster addressed were met with denial from city, state, and federal agencies. However, after advocacy efforts for over a decade, Congress passed the James Zadroga 9/11 Health and Compensation Act in 2010 and reauthorized it in 2015. Their chapter offers insight into health-related trauma resulting from the attacks; responses of governmental entities at local, state, and national levels; and the mobilization of individuals and groups in response to various challenges, some of which continue today. The chapter concludes by describing what we can learn from the post–9/11 health crisis and by identifying emerging 9/11 health-related issues.

In "Posttraumatic Stress Disorder Following 9/11: What We Know Now," Ari Lowell, Ariel Durosky, Anne Hilburn, Liat Helpman, Xi Zhu, and Yuval Neria discuss posttraumatic stress disorder (PTSD), the largest category of mental health issues that emerged after the September 11 World Trade Center attacks. The authors describe the nature of PTDS and, based on an updated review of the epidemiological literature, describe its prevalence among groups directly exposed to 9/11, how the expression of PTSD changed over time, and associated risk factors. They find that while rates of PTSD decreased over time for most high exposure groups (i.e., those living or working in close proximity to 9/11), rates increased for first responders and rescue/recovery workers, with some differences between traditional (i.e., police officers, firemen) and nontraditional (i.e., civilian) responders. The authors observe that some 9/11 populations were understudied and that longitudinal data on youth is quite limited.

In "Living in Houses Without Walls: Muslim Youth in New York City in the Aftermath of 9/11," Diala Shamas describes how, in the immediate aftermath of September 11, the New York City Police Department (NYPD) embarked on an expansive program to surveil New York City's large, diverse, and overwhelmingly immigrant Muslim American community. As leaked NYPD documents reveal, this elaborate, secret surveillance program mapped, monitored, and analyzed American Muslim daily life throughout New York City with a special focus on Muslim students. Drawing on the author's interviews with targeted college students, this chapter describes some of the devastating impacts of this program of surveillance on Muslim youth.

Finally, in "Memory, Site, and Object: The September 11 Memorial Museum," Susan Opotow and Karyna Pryiomka describe the design and development of the September 11 Memorial Museum at the World Trade Center site from the perspective of architect Mark Wagner of Davis Brody

Bond, whose work on the museum, which began in 2004, was preceded by his work at Ground Zero archiving significant objects in the debris left by the Twin Towers' collapse. The museum opened in 2014 with the goal of bearing witness to the 1993 and 2001 terrorist attacks on the World Trade Center site and honoring victims of those attacks, those who risked their lives to save others, and the thousands of survivors. Wagner describes the principles guiding the design of the museum and the challenges of this work. The authors discuss the museum's design, development, and artifacts in light of psychological, materialist, and museum studies on perception and emotion. Doing so clarifies how the site enables visitors to experience the significance and emotion of the site and connect with a traumatic past.

## Conclusion

*New York After 9/11* offers insightful, poignant, and critical observations about the way that New Yorkers and the City as a whole responded to and coped with September 11, 2001's aftermath. The chapters clarify that recovery from 9/11 has been a long and braided process that unfolded in different ways in different spheres. The book's chapters reveal the importance of collaborative efforts, tenacity over time, and the value of community voice, inclusion, and transparency.

As time passes, New York's recovery from 9/11 will become increasingly less obvious as it fades from foreground to background, but this process is clearly not done. As 9/11 shifts from memory to history, *New York After 9/11* analyzes significant challenges, conflicts, and changes that emerged. Looking back on the aftermath of this traumatic and destructive event offers readers, scholars, and policymakers deeper insight into the past so that we can learn from it as we move forward.

### Notes

1. *The 9/11 Commission Report* (2004). Available at https://goo.gl/Lm8Sdb.
2. Sorkin, Zukin, and Zukin, 2002; see also "Conflict and Change: New York City's Rebirth After 9/11" in this book.
3. Silver, 2011.
4. Kirschenblatt-Gimblett, 2003, has a rich account of the post–9/11 period; see also Belmonte and Opotow, 2017, for a description of the creation of the September 11 Digital Archive.
5. Smith, 2006.
6. Chernick, 2005.
7. US Bureau of Labor Statistics, "Extended Mass Layoffs and the 9/11 Attacks," September 10, 2003: https://goo.gl/5zy6bp.

8. Low, 2004; Chin 2005.

9. Wallace, 2002.

10. Sagalyn, 2006.

11. Low, 2004; Low, Taplin, and Lamb, 2005; Fullilove, Hernandez-Cordero, Stevens Madoff, and Fullilove, 2004; Smithsimon, 2011.

12. See "Health Impacts of 9/11" in this book.

13. Young, 2017.

14. "Little Syria: New York City's Forgotten Arab-American Neighborhood," *Daily News*, n.d.; Alexandra S. Levin, "A Lost Little Syria," *New York Times*, May 24, 2016.

15. David W. Dunlap, "When an Arab Enclave Thrived Downtown," *New York Times*, August 24, 2010; David W. Dunlap, "Little Syria (Now Tiny Syria) Finds New Advocates," *New York Times*, January 1, 2012.

16. Yamin, 1998.

17. Berlin and Harris, 2005.

18. Kirshenblatt-Gimblett, 2003.

19. See "Memory Foundations" in this book.

20. David W. Dunlap, "At Ground Zero, Scenes from the Ice Age," *New York Times*, September 21, 2008.

21. Laura Ly, "Researchers: Centuries-Old Ship at NYC Ground Zero Likely from Philadelphia," CNN.com, August 6, 2014: https://goo.gl/NL1cSg; see also "Pieces of Ship Made in 1700s Found at Ground Zero Building Site," also available at CNN.com.

22. Smithsonian Institution, "Manahatta to Manhattan: Native Americans in Lower Manhattan." Available at https://goo.gl/ekxBNX.

23. Snejana Farberov, "How Hurricane Sandy Flooded New York back to Its 17th Century Shape as It Inundated 400 Years of Reclaimed Land," *Daily Mail*, June 16, 2013.

24. Editorial, "Hurricane Sandy's Rising Costs," *New York Times*, November 27, 2012.

25. Farberov, "How Hurricane Sandy Flooded New York."

26. See "Living in Houses Without Walls: Muslim Youth in New York City in the Aftermath of 9/11" in this book; see also Shamas and Arastu, 2013.

27. See "Health Impacts of 9/11" in this book; Nordgrén, Goldstein, and Izeman, 2002; Newman, 2013; Office of the Inspector General, 2003.

28. See "Urban Security in NYC Post–9/11: Risk and Realities" in this book.

29. See "Health Impacts of 9/11" in this book.

## References

9/11 Commission. *The 9/11 Commission Report: Final Report of the National Commission on Terrorist Attacks Upon the United States*. New York: Norton, 2011.

Belmonte, Kimberly, and Susan Opotow. "Archivists on Archives and Social Justice." *Qualitative Psychology* 4, no. 1 (2017): 58.

Berlin, Ira, and Leslie M. Harris. *Slavery in New York*. New York: New Press, 2005.

Chernick, Howard, ed. *Resilient City: The Economic Impact of 9/11*. New York: Russell Sage Foundation, 2005.

Chin, Margaret M. "Moving On: Chinese Garment Workers after 9/11." *Wounded City: The Social Impact of 9/11* (2005): 184–207.

Fullilove, Mindy Thompson, Lourdes Hernandez-Cordero, Jennifer Stevens Madoff, and Robert E. Fullilove III. "Promoting Collective Recovery through Organizational Mobilization: The Post–9/11 Disaster Relief Work of NYC Recovers." *Journal of Biosocial Science* 36, no. 4 (2004): 479–489.

Kirschenblatt-Gimblett, Barbara. "Kodak Moments, Flashbulb Memories: Reflections on 9/11." *The Drama Review* 47, no. 1 (2003): 11–48.

Low, Setha M., Dana H. Taplin, and Mike Lamb. "Battery Park City: An Ethnographic Field Study of the Community Impact of 9/11." *Urban Affairs Review* 40, no. 5 (2005): 655–682.

Low, Setha M. "The Memorialization of September 11: Dominant and Local Discourses on the Rebuilding of the World Trade Center Site." *American Ethnologist* 31, no. 3 (2004): 326–339.

Newman, David M. *Protecting Worker and Community Health: Are We Prepared for the Next 9/11?* New York, NY: New York Committee for Occupational Safety and Health (NYCOSH), December 30, 2013. Accessed December 29, 2017. https://goo.gl/jxKV5B.

Nordgrén, Megan D., Eric A. Goldstein, and Mark A. Izeman. *The Environmental Impacts of the World Trade Center Attacks: A Preliminary Assessment*. Washington, DC: Natural Resources Defense Council, 2002.

Office of the Inspector General. *EPA's Response to the World Trade Center Collapse: Challenges, Successes, and Areas for Improvement*. Washington DC: United States Environmental Protection Agency, 2003.

Sagalyn, Lynne B. *Power at Ground Zero: Politics, Money, and the Remaking of Lower Manhattan*. New York: Oxford University Press, 2016.

Shamas, Diala, and Nermeen Arastu. "Mapping Muslims: NYPD Spying and Its Impact on American Muslims." New York: 2013. Available at https://goo.gl/jxyXcy.

Shulan, Michael, Gilles Peress, Alice Rose George, and Charles Traub. *Here Is New York: A Democracy of Photographs*. New York: Scalo, 2002.

Silver, Roxane Cohen. "An Introduction to '9/11: Ten Years Later.'" *American Psychologist* 66, no. 6 (2011): 427.

Smithsimon, Gregory. *September 12: Community and Neighborhood Recovery at Ground Zero*. New York: New York University Press, 2011.

Smith, Terry E. *The Architecture of Aftermath*. Chicago: University of Chicago Press, 2006.

Sorkin, Michael, Michael Zukin, and Sharon Zukin. *After the World Trade Center: Rethinking New York City*. New York: Routledge, 2002.

Sweeney, Patrick, and Susan Opotow. "'Why There?' Islamophobia, Environmental Conflict, and Justice at Ground Zero." *Social Justice Research* 26, no. 4
(2013): 492–512.

Wallace, Mike. *A New Deal for New York*. New York: Bell & Weiland, 2002.

Yamin, Rebecca. "Lurid Tales and Homely Stories of New York's Notorious
Five Points." *Historical Archaeology* 32, no. 1 (1998): 74–85.

Young, Michelle. "Radio Row: A Tinkerer's Paradise and Makerspace, Lost
to the World Trade Center." *6sqft*, September 25, 2017: https://goo.gl/
CTg1eH.

# Conflict and Change
## New York City's Rebirth after 9/11

Zachary Baron Shemtob, Patrick Sweeney,
and Susan Opotow

**9/11** was a world-historical event. It is therefore of little surprise that so much attention has been paid to its impact on American society and global affairs. What has been less studied is 9/11's direct impact on those persons most directly affected by the World Trade Center's destruction: the residents of New York City and Lower Manhattan. By using *New York Times* articles as data, this chapter surveys the lived experiences of New Yorkers in 9/11's aftermath, focused in particular on the five years that followed this horrifying event and the 2010 controversy surrounding the so-called Ground Zero Mosque.

We begin this chapter by sketching out how scholars have defined the concept of a disaster and the idea that, in a disaster's wake, a community resumes its prior equilibrium or adapts to a new one.[1] We then identify various priorities that consumed post–9/11 New Yorkers, noting how some of these priorities quickly came into conflict. Specifically, we found that New Yorkers were initially concerned with whether life would return to normal, before shifting their focus to concerns over the physical rebuilding process and the political struggles that such recovery entailed. We then compare these findings with the controversy over the so-called Ground Zero Mosque several years later. Finally, we describe a new equilibrium that emerged among New Yorkers directly and indirectly affected by 9/11, which is still being shaped to this day.

## Understanding Disaster

American sociologists began systematically studying disasters during World War II through military-funded research that focused on civilian populations' response to large-scale bombings.[2] Disaster research accelerated in the 1950s when the National Academy of Sciences National Research Council began supporting research on large-scale natural and technological crises.[3] Despite six decades of research on populations' responses to disasters,[4] sociologists continue to develop and debate the meaning of the term "disaster."[5]

Perhaps Charles Fritz's 1961 definition of disaster remains the most prominent as an event "in which a society, or a relatively self-sufficient subdivision of a society, undergoes several dangers and incurs such loses to its members and physical appurtenances that the social structure is disrupted and the fulfillment of all or some of the essential functions of the society is prevented."[6] According to Fritz, disasters inevitably: (1) threaten biological survival, including subsistence, shelter, and health; (2) disrupt the normal order of things, including a society's divisions of labor, authority patterns, cultural norms, and social roles; (3) threaten values, shared definitions of reality, and communication mechanisms; and (4) modify motivations within social and cultural systems. Elaborating on Fritz's definition, Russell Dynes identified seven central elements of disaster: (1) an event (2) located in time and space (3) in which a community (4) undergoes severe danger (5) and incurs losses (6) so that the social structure is disrupted (7) and the fulfillment of all or some of its essential functions is prevented.[7]

Stanley Cohen has additionally focused on how disasters disrupt the normal order of things.[8] According to Cohen, after such events a "community either recovers its former equilibrium or achieves a stable adaptation to the changes which the disaster may have brought about."[9] Kai Erikson has further explored this idea.[10] After studying a disastrous flood at Buffalo Creek, West Virginia, Erikson concluded that persons affected by disaster undergo (1) the sense that the disaster will never end; (2) the feeling of vulnerability from having lost a sense of immunity to misfortune; (3) a changed sense of oneself, including how one relates to others; and (4) a changed view of the world that now includes a sense of life's utter precariousness. Erikson, like Cohen, argues that it is not disaster, per se, that leads to change, but it is "how *people react to them* rather than *what they are* that give [such] events whatever traumatic quality they can be said to have" (italics in original).[11]

## September 11 in the *New York Times*

Few disasters in United States history compare to the 9/11 attacks, which affected communities throughout the country and the globe. This event took the lives of passengers and crew aboard four hijacked airplanes in New York City; Arlington, Virginia; and Shanksville, Pennsylvania; workers and visitors at the World Trade Center; military personnel at the Pentagon; and people who later died from exposure to toxic wreckage resulting from the attacks.[12] But of the almost 3,000 fatalities that resulted from the attacks on New York City and Washington DC on 9/11, most (93 percent, over 2,800 deaths) occurred in a single community, Lower Manhattan.[13]

Post-disaster 9/11 scholarship concerning New York City has largely focused on (1) the short-term dynamics at the macro level, as the city as a whole moved from shock to solidarity;[14] (2) the longer-term dynamics focused at the individual level, particularly individual bereavement, trauma, and PTSD;[15] (3) Islamophobic bias and violence directed at people perceived to be Middle Eastern, Arab, or Muslim;[16] and (4) evaluations of technical aspects of the 9/11 attacks from the perspective of specific professions, such as technology, security, and mental health.[17] Far fewer studies have focused, as we do, on the years-long trajectory of this tragic event in the lives of New Yorkers after 9/11.

## Researching Post–9/11 New York City

To study how New Yorkers responded to the events of 9/11, we worked from an archive of *New York Times* articles that one of us (Opotow) gathered from September 2001 until five years later when stories of everyday New Yorkers' responses to 9/11 became less prominent in the news. These news articles offer unparalleled insight into the immediate aftermath of 9/11 and provide information on those affected by the attacks, and how the attack impacted everyday lives in many different spheres of society. We recognize that such articles are not free of bias, as people with fewer resources and who do not affect the flow of profits and corporate agendas may get less attention in the news.[18] And, as we discuss in the following section, media interest in once-newsworthy topics fades dramatically over time.[19] Nevertheless, after 9/11, newspapers offered unparalleled access into New Yorkers' immediate and long-term responses to this event. Specifically, the *New York Times*, a newspaper of record with a long-established reputation for meeting high journalistic standards,[20] devoted significant space to New York City and Lower Manhattan in the aftermath of 9/11, offering rich and detailed accounts of 9/11 and its effects on the city.

To conduct this study, we first constructed an archive of *New York Times* articles focusing on the aftermath of the World Trade Center attacks in New York City. By the three-year mark, we had collected more than three thousand articles. By 2006 this topic became less frequent in the news, and we therefore decided that this was a natural stopping point. Working alongside research assistants,[21] we sorted the articles from this five-year period using an iterative process of coding, discussing, and recoding the articles to create a set of categories encompassing diverse topics and levels of analysis, from individuals to neighborhoods, institutions, agencies, and the city as a whole. Prominent categories included: fear of terrorism, rescue and recovery, changes in routines, death, health, injury, economic loss, the families of people who died, the victim compensation fund, replacing the World Trade Center, rescue and recovery crews, economic impacts, Lower Manhattan restoration and redevelopment, emerging memorials, and 9/11 in the arts. Based on this, we ultimately developed a set of six overarching categories: (1) compensation; (2) World Trade Center rebirth; (3) narratives about everyday lives; (4) fear, health, and quality of life; (5) emerging memorials around the world; and (6) artistic works on 9/11.

For this chapter, we report on one category, World Trade Center rebirth. This category centers on New York City's journey from damage to regeneration, reporting on how New Yorkers sought to recover in 9/11's aftermath and how this was understood and enacted at the personal and civic levels. It thus offers a nuanced and unique account of the physical, psychological, and civic challenge New Yorkers faced as they sought to rebuild their own lives as well as the World Trade Center site (dubbed "Ground Zero") and lower Manhattan.[22]

Replicating the collaborative and interactive process used in our initial coding of all the articles, we identified eight subcategories for World Trade Center rebirth:

1. Professional/architectural planning ($n = 176$): Articles dealing with professionals (other than politicians) directly involved with rebuilding the World Trade Center, including the buildings, landscape, and urban design surrounding this project.
2. Political issues ($n = 131$): Articles describing the political climate that emerged in the rebuilding process. These focused on specific political figures (e.g., mayors, governors, senators, etc.) and political struggles at city, state, and federal levels that arose over various projects.
3. Business/economy ($n = 94$): Articles focusing on the rebuilding of New York City's economic infrastructure, the reopening of

restaurants and retail stores, the revival of tourism, and financial aid from the state and government to businesses and industries.

4. Return to normality ($n=83$): Articles focusing on New Yorkers attempt to recover from 9/11 while also recognizing that their lives had irrevocably changed.

5. Citizen participation in planning ($n=65$): Articles focused on public participation in the rebuilding process.

6. Sadness/melancholy ($n=33$): Articles focusing on New Yorkers' emotional trauma, sadness, and sense of paralysis, as well as articles recounting how individuals, communities, and organizations had difficulty functioning optimally or moving forward after 9/11.

7. Cleanup ($n=19$): Articles focusing on the removal of bodies from the World Trade Center site, the discovery of bone fragments and personal items in the debris, and health hazards resulting from the World Trade Center's collapse.

8. Progress and deadlines ($n=16$): Articles focusing on the disparities between project completion dates and progress on the ground.

We then charted the frequencies of these eight categories using 30 percent as a viable cutoff point to designate dominant categories for each year (see Appendix A). The most dominant categories that emerged were: return to normality (33 percent, 2001), business/economy (31 percent, 2001), professional/architectural planning (31 percent, 43 percent, and 40 percent, 2002–2004 respectively), and politics (44 percent and 42 percent, 2005–2006 respectively). Interestingly, we also found that the dominant categories shifted over these five years. The next section describes these findings year by year.

## Year by Year: World Trade Center Rebirth

*2001: Return to Normality and Business-Economic Recovery*

In the fifteen weeks after September 11, we found that return to normality and business/economy were the dominant categories in newspaper articles focused on the rebirth of the World Trade Center. Indeed, almost two-thirds of the articles during this time centered on these two categories. Initially, the desire to return to normality was the most prevalent category. This category rapidly declined, however, with most such articles occurring in the first few weeks (Week 1 = 11; Week 2 = 13; Week 3 = 12; Week 4 = 5; subsequent weeks = 1). Thus, this was a topic of intense but ultimately fleeting concern, a change we analyze in greater depth in the following subsection.

The other major category to emerge after 9/11 focused on business and the economy. In the fifteen weeks following 9/11, one to two articles per week were published on this topic. These articles largely featured themes of resilience, as businesses attempted to bounce back and move forward despite damages, challenges, and the social and economic upheaval caused by 9/11. Indeed, each move forward was often portrayed as a victory or a symbol of New Yorkers' defiance against their attackers. As we describe in the next section, many business-focused articles in 2001 specifically related to entertainment as an indicator of New York City's recovery, resilience, resourcefulness, and vitality.

*2002–2004: Professionals/Architectural Planning*

Professional/architectural planning was the dominant category for the rebuilding process for three years, from 2002 to 2004. In 2002, these articles centered on competing visions for constructing the Ground Zero site; downtown's redevelopment and restoration; and the selection of consultants and design teams for the project as a whole and for specific elements of the redevelopment process. In 2003, conflict first began to emerge over how to how to reshape downtown and who should do it. Many articles here discussed professionals and architectural planning for rebuilding the Ground Zero site and appraisals of the proposed designs. In particular, the articles featured architects David Childs and Daniel Libeskind and their competing visions of redevelopment of the World Trade Center site. In 2004, conflicts among architects, politicians, and the leaseholder, Larry Silverstein, were especially prominent in the news.

*2005–2006: Political Issues*

For the fourth and fifth years after the 9/11 attacks, political issues came to the fore. These articles included: politicians vying to lead the rebuilding effort; the complex approval process for the Trade Center rail hub; controversies concerning the Freedom Museum; Mayor Michael Bloomberg's vision for rebuilding; the reconsidering of prior building plans; the collision between design and expense; the unclear role of oversight agencies; and the selection of a joint venture in order to build the PATH rail station.

In 2006, news articles on the rebirth of the World Trade Center focused on the allocation of post–9/11 funds; the clash over redevelopment of the Ground Zero site between US Senator Charles Schumer and Mayor Bloomberg; New York Governor George Pataki's attempts to revive talks on construction and his dealings with World Trade Center Leaseholder Larry Silverstein; summits convened to discuss Ground Zero plans; the resignation of the memorial chief at Ground Zero; disputes over World Trade Center tenant deals; and plans by the United States and New York State governmental agencies to occupy Freedom Tower.

## Analysis: Shifting Concerns, Conflicts, and Challenges, 2001–2006

The preceding discussion identified the shifting terrain and a variety of challenges and conflicts in the five years following 9/11. A deeper analysis also found that five key themes emerged over this time in (loosely) sequential order, which we explore in this section. The shifting dominance of these challenges and concerns reveals complex tensions set in motion after the World Trade Center's destruction.

### Theme One: Normality and Change

As described in the previous section, in 9/11's immediate aftermath, the news first concerned peoples' desire for things to get back to normal. The shock of 9/11 prompted existential and practical questions: What does it mean for things to be normal? Will normality return by resuming one's routine daily activities and social relations? Or is something else necessary, such as rebuilding what has been lost? And does returning to normality ultimately disrespect those who were killed?

In the weeks after 9/11, news articles traced different ways of resuming normality from small everyday activities like sketching or eating salad in the park[23] to taking part in larger social events such as movies and football games.[24] In these articles, people prized what had been familiar and taken for granted, and they found a sense of mastery, even triumph, in doing what previously had been routine.

Too much normality, however, was also seen as problematic.[25] For example, New Yorkers questioned such basic things as whether it was okay to laugh, or whether this was inappropriate given recent events. Individuals consequently wondered what matters were frivolous and thereby possibly a misguided preoccupation, or whether embracing some frivolity was helpful to dispel a sense of despair, fear, or helplessness.[26] These articles reported that New Yorkers were continually plagued by such questions but very few of the articles (or personal narratives) provided any answers.

*Theme Two: Entertainment and Solidarity*

A second theme that emerged in the *New York Times* articles in 2002 was the connection between solidarity and popular entertainment. Immediately after the attack, the city lacked reliable communication and transportation networks, increasing individuals' sense of isolation and anxiety. As theaters, sports events, nightclubs, and museums reopened one by one, the news cheered the return of the liveliness they contributed to a beleaguered city.

Although these destinations offered distraction, perhaps more important, they allowed people to be closer to one another. Indeed, these communal events engendered a sense of camaraderie even when those gathered had little in common besides having lived through the experience of 9/11.[27] Initially, media executives assumed that the collective psyche would be easily offended, frightened, or traumatized by violent entertainment.[28] But regardless of such content, cultural events seemed to distract, soothe, and alleviate persons' boredom, dread, and repetitive thoughts.[29]

Initially, news articles principally focused on the public's return to such venues. Over time, however, the articles began focusing on cultural practitioners themselves. Various jazz musicians, for example, were featured as describing their reluctance to leave their family or even play music.[30] Other entertainers expressed caution about evoking audience sensitivities, memories, and fears connected with September 11.[31] Performers also attempted to "carry on in ways large and small," organizing blood drives or volunteering to take part in ongoing rescue operations at Ground Zero.[32]

Interestingly, as detailed in the previous section, this emphasis on entertainment faded from the news early in 2002, only a few months after 9/11. At this point, news articles concerned the architecture and design competitions surrounding Ground Zero,[33] and by 2003, these competitions became a public spectacle in themselves, pitting particular designers and their advocates, often prominent politicians, against one another.[34]

*Theme Three: Socioemotional Versus Economic Concerns*

A third sequential theme was the struggle between socioemotional and economic values, which became evident as people looked ahead to the rebuilding of the World Trade Center site in 2002. Social psychologist Morton Deutsch has observed that socioemotional and economic values inevitably conflict. The former focuses on the "solidarity relations among group members," and the latter on "external tasks" and "problem solving."[35] In other words, as journalist Alan Murray has suggested, commemorating loss and accruing capital may constitute discrete and potentially opposed societal priorities.[36]

This tension between these value systems emerged in 2002 in lower Manhattan when designs for the new World Trade Center site raised fears that a purely commercial building would disrespect those who had died.[37] Indeed, the six earliest designs of the new World Trade Center embodied this fear: These designs were vehemently opposed by the public not for aesthetic or functional reasons, but due to the large proportion of space allocated for offices.[38] As a victim's relative remarked, "we got what was there before,"[39] apparently disappointed by the replication of the original World Trade Center's commercial purpose along with its utilitarianism and (assumed) lack of heart.

Perhaps remarkably, these criticisms resulted in a quick shift by city and state officials. The Lower Manhattan Development Corporation, for example, which had endorsed the original six designs, agreed to reduce and revise these proposals.[40] The six designs in the initial competition were then scrapped in favor of a new public competition and revisions to the process that would make it less opaque.[41] The next set of designs garnered more public approval, but the public's response to them was mixed. Nikki Stern, whose husband had been killed on 9/11, lamented that this round of designs "involved a lot more design and creativity," but did not yet reconcile how to balance commemorating the lives of those who died with the goal of commercial development.[42]

We thus see the emergence of two issues here. First is the supposed heartlessness and depersonalization of economic decision making, which is driven by the bottom line rather than a concern for suffering and loss. The interests of developers and businessmen were in stark contrast with what the families of those killed on 9/11 and what the larger public saw as an appropriate memorial.[43] The second issue is an ironic refutation of what the original World Trade Center actually stood for: to foster trade on a global scale and incorporate a significant amount of office space in order to do so. In other words, the World Trade Center epitomized "hard economics."[44] In contrast, the same site post–9/11 was being held to a higher standard. Unlike the original World Trade Center, the new site was expected to transcend business interests and the cold agglomeration of capital to attend instead to social relations and the commemoration of loss.

*Theme Four: The Fading Public Voice*

A fourth theme that emerged in the World Trade Center's rebirth was the role of the public voice and its eventual disappearance. The salience of the public voice can be traced throughout all five years after 9/11. Neverthe-less, as explained in the previous section, public influence reached its apex in 2002 and 2003—in the early part of the design process—before being displaced in the news by attention to various political leaders.

Immediately after 9/11, the *New York Times* featured a multiplicity of dif-ferent voices, from affected downtown street vendors to victims' spouses.[45] At first, no voice was treated by the *New York Times* as paramount, and thus no person or group was seen as speaking for the public as a whole. Rather, the public was viewed as united in its shock, grief, and desire to resume normality.

As decisions about the rebuilding process gained ascendency, how-ever, this sense of solidarity and egalitarianism faded and victims' families held the greatest sway. Wives of those who perished on 9/11 were most prominently featured in the news, with their grief seen as providing a moral clarity that transcended petty politics or individual self-interest.[46] But, by the middle of 2003 even the voices of victims' families were ef-fectively sidelined. Certain persons from the public (e.g., survivors or vic-tim's family members) were selected for some planning committees or commissions and their voices were occasionally mentioned in the news.[47] Nonetheless, the *New York Times* principally focused on prominent indi-viduals tasked with the site's rebuilding, whether Governor George Pataki or architects Daniel Libeskind and David Childs.[48] As the process became enmeshed in negotiations and political maneuvering and the focus moved to questions of logistics and technical expertise, the public voice became less and less prominent.

*Theme Five: Priorities and Power*

The final major theme we found to emerge in the 9/11 rebuilding pro-cess was, unsurprisingly, power. The city remained relatively peaceful following 9/11, with little looting or violence. At first, shocked political leaders appeared to offer the public little more than avuncular advice such as to "go to the theater."[49]

As we described above, however, in 2003 and beyond political dynam-ics took center stage in Lower Manhattan. Conflicts erupted over dueling design conceptions for the new World Trade Center site, as politicians aligned themselves with particular architects and became champions of specific visions for Ground Zero.[50] This was further complicated by the interests of the World Trade Center's leaseholder, Larry Silverstein; the Port Authority of New York and New Jersey, the site's owner; the Lower Manhattan Development Corporation, which had administrative control over the World Trade Center site; New York State Governor George Pataki; and New York City Mayor Michael Bloomberg.[51]

Eventually, the initial hopes for a simple consensus gave way to more coercive methods to resolve intransigent conflicts, such as when Governor Pataki declared a midnight deadline for the disputing parties to reach agreement.[52] Such tactics effectively eliminated public input and attempted to force more powerful individuals to compromise on their preferred rebuilding goals. Although eliminating transparency and public engagement may have expedited the rebuilding process, it also may have prevented other issues from being raised by a broader set of stakeholders with a range of interests in the World Trade Center site.[53]

## The Park51 Controversy

Although the preceding five themes emerged in the half-decade following 9/11, it was unclear, without further inquiry, whether they remained germane as the post-disaster period later unfolded. To determine whether such issues persisted beyond 2006, we therefore focused on another event directly linked with 9/11 that generated a significant amount of news coverage: a highly-publicized controversy in 2010 surrounding the development of Park51 in Lower Manhattan, the so-called Ground Zero Mosque. In the following section we describe this controversy, discuss the five themes analyzed in the previous section and their relevance to this event, and, to further broaden our understanding of post–9/11 conflict and change, compare how these themes manifested themselves in the first five years after 9/11 versus in the debate over Park51.

### A Brief History of Park51

Although the Park51 Islamic Community Center was known to many as the "Ground Zero Mosque," it is neither at Ground Zero nor is it technically a mosque. Consequently, we use its official name, Park51. The site consists of two adjacent buildings located at 45–47 Park Place and 49–51 Park Place between Church Street and West Broadway in Lower Manhattan, two blocks (600 feet or 180 meters) north of the World Trade Center site.[54]

Modeled on the 92nd Street Y, a nonprofit cultural and community center in Manhattan, Park51 was originally named "Cordoba House" and planned as an interfaith community center open to all New Yorkers, regardless of religion. Park51's planners wanted its thirteen stories to "rise two blocks from the pit of dust and cranes where the twin towers once stood, a symbol of the resilience of the American melting pot."[55] They initially envisioned a building with two floors for Muslim prayer space. Other floors would house a five-hundred-seat auditorium, a theater, a performing arts center, a fitness center, a swimming pool, a basketball court, a childcare center, an art gallery, a bookstore, a culinary school, and a restaurant.[56]

The center's construction was first reported as controversial in the *New York Times* in May 2010, when a normally uneventful community board meeting turned into a raucous hearing debating whether a supposed mosque should be built at Ground Zero.[57] This conflict over the two buildings' proposed usage soon erupted into a media firestorm driven by anti-Muslim groups and politicians who seized on this controversy. Although many New Yorkers were appalled by what they saw as the Islamophobic views concerning Park51, some also expressed reservations about building an Islamic cultural center so close to Ground Zero.[58]

After media attention to the controversy diminished and the development plans cleared the normal regulatory hurdles, construction on Park51 began. Nevertheless, new obstacles to the project soon emerged. In 2011, a rift developed between Park51's developer, Sharif El-Gamal, and the imam associated with the project, Feisal Abdul Rauf. El-Gamal and Rauf clashed over the future of the project, leading Rauf to eventually step down, only to have his replacement resign three weeks later for making homophobic remarks.[59] Meanwhile, on September 21, 2011, a surprisingly quiet and controversy-free photo exhibit marked the official launch of Park51 in a makeshift gallery space on the ground floor of 45–47 Park Place.[60]

Nevertheless, Park51's troubles persisted. Later that year, the landlord of one of the buildings, Consolidated Edison, demanded $1.7 million in back rent from the developer, initiating a dispute that further endangered the proposed plans.[61] After the rent dispute was resolved, ongoing fundraising shortfalls plagued the project.[62] As this is being written (January 2018), plans for the site now consist of luxury apartments ranging in price from approximately $2 to 41 million.[63] Ultimately, this forty-three-story apartment complex is expected to open in 2019 alongside a much scaled-down three-story Islamic museum and public plaza.[64]

*Thematic Analysis of the Park51 Controversy*

NORMALITY AND CHANGE
As described in the prior section, in the first five years after 9/11, the theme of normality and change was reflected in the tension between

persons' desires to return to normal while appropriately honoring the memory of those lost. By 2009, New Yorkers had eight years to resume their lives. Perhaps for this reason, the early plans to develop Park51 were not controversial. Indeed, they drew "encouragement from city officials and the surrounding neighborhood," with a spokesman for the mayor quoted as saying "If it's legal, the building owners have a right to do what they want."[65]

This sense of civic calm was not to last, however. Five months later, stoked by Internet commentators and right-wing websites, Lower Manhattan's Community Board No. 1 was inundated with calls and emails concerning the proposal, the majority of these from outside New York City.[66] Consequently, the community board hearing that followed erupted into a four-hour heated debate over the appropriateness of the plans, between those who claimed the community center would represent a beacon of tolerance and those who claimed that it would offend the memories of the persons killed on 9/11.[67]

As local questions of neighborhood planning were transformed into national and international debates on the nature of Islam and the legacy of 9/11, New Yorkers were therefore thrust back into the meaning of the attacks and away from ordinary questions of city administration and bureaucracy. Although certain New Yorkers believed the "Ground Zero Mosque" was an affront to those killed by Islamic terrorists, other New Yorkers were nonplussed by the plans and saw the opposition as amounting to "hysteria."[68] They emphasized that the neighborhood had long included a storefront mosque and also had such disreputable institutions as "a strip joint, a porno store and a government-run bookie operation."[69] Because of the Park51 controversy, New Yorkers once again scrutinized normal patterns of urban life and varied kinds of social activities for their ethical significance. Thus, people were forced to grapple with what was right to do in the "sacred ground" surrounding Ground Zero, and what routines of life would permanently alter as a result of 9/11.

ENTERTAINMENT AND SOLIDARITY

During the first five years, the theme of solidarity and entertainment was illustrated by articles discussing the public's return to cultural and social events before shifting to a focus on the public spectacle of design competitions themselves. The controversy over Park51 provided a similar spectacle. What could have been a local decision regarding the approval and development of a cultural institution by a community board was transformed into an uproar and media sensation virtually overnight. As opponents of Park51's supporters became louder, various right-wing politicians and anti-Muslim groups increasingly made media headlines, from Pamela Geller, the founder of an Islamophobic website and the Stop Islamization of America/the American Freedom Defense Initiative,[70] to the pastor of a small Florida church who threatened to burn copies of the Koran.[71] For many people living in New York City, the controversy was galling. An analysis of the news articles on Park51 in that period found that many New Yorkers, particularly those who lived close to the site, were not likely to oppose its construction and viewed the opposition as antithetical to the inclusionary ethos embedded in what they viewed as New York values and American ideals.[72]

Interestingly, each side relied on a sense of collective solidarity to legitimate its cause. Many of those who supported Park51, like Mayor Bloomberg, appealed to an abstract notion of "American values," arguing that moving the site would insult American Muslims and damage the nation's standing.[73] Those opposed appealed to a vision of America under siege. Pamela Geller positioned Park51 as a sign of Islamic ideological encroachment on American soil,[74] illustrated in advertisements she submitted to the New York City Metropolitan Transit Authority for display on city buses that linked Park51 to the 9/11 attacks by calling it the "WTC Mega Mosque."[75] Meanwhile, politicians like Ilario Pantano, a Republican candidate for the US House of Representatives in North Carolina, campaigned on the Park51 conflict, claiming that it "stirred voters in his rural district hundreds of miles away from Ground Zero."[76] Although both sides appealed to America's collective identity, they therefore did so by advocating for entirely different outcomes and articulating differing conceptions of American priorities, ideals, and identity.

SOCIOEMOTIONAL VS. ECONOMIC CONCERNS

In the first five years, the theme of socioemotional versus economic concerns reflected the tension and conflict that emerged between an emphasis on the economic bottom line versus memorialization of 9/11. This theme was also manifest in the Park51 controversy with the eventual eclipse of economic concerns as advocates and critics of Park51 appealed to socioemotional concerns. Opponents argued that the center should not be built because the World Trade Center included not only the "the immediate buildings, but large swaths around them that . . . aren't measured in meters or yards, but in emotional sparks."[77] Proponents, like Mayor Michael Bloomberg's "voice began to crack" as he spoke for the importance of religious freedom as a core American value.[78]

Besides the public controversy, the tension between socioemotional and economic concerns also played out in the rift between the project's developer, El-Gamal, and its religious leader, Imam Rauf. The two ultimately disagreed over the project's size, its commercial nature, and whether it should primarily appeal to Muslims or all religious groups.[79] Whereas El-Gamal particularly stressed Park51's economic potential, Rauf principally sought to create a viable community center.[80] Their disagreement eventually led to Rauf's stepping down, and El-Gamal coming to prioritize Park51's real estate potential. In 2017, the revised plans for Park51's cultural and religious spaces shifted from a thirteen-story community center with prayer space and public event spaces to a forty-three-story apartment tower with multimillion-dollar luxury apartments and a scaled-down three-story Islamic museum and public plaza next door.[81]

THE FADING PUBLIC VOICE

The Park51 controversy, from its inception, involved a mixture of positions and voices. The *New York Times* commissioned a poll of New Yorkers' views on the subject and found that two-thirds of participants wanted the site relocated to a less "controversial" area.[82] Family members of those lost on 9/11 were also portrayed as "weigh[ing] in" against the project.[83] Park51 was described, for example, by Sally Regenhard, the mother of a firefighter who died on 9/11, as "sacrilege on sacred ground."[84] At one point, an ex-firefighter gained prominence after (unsuccessfully) suing to give landmark protection to the site in order to prevent Park51 from being built there.[85]

Ultimately, however, politicians and other prominent public figures from both sides of the issue dominated the conversation over Park51, like that over the rebirth of the World Trade Center. These included Mayor Bloomberg (for), New York State Assembly Speaker Sheldon Silver (against), New York State gubernatorial candidates Rick Lazio and Carl Paladino (both against), US President Barack Obama (for), former US Speaker of the House Newt Gingrich (against), US vice presidential nominee Sarah Palin (against), the Koran-burning pastor Terry Jones (against), the Dutch politician Geert Wilders (against), and the aforementioned congressional candidate Ilario Pantano and prominent anti-Muslim blogger Pamela Geller (both against).[86] As these prominent voices came to dominate the news coverage, they acted as stand-ins for the public at large. Thus, whereas Gingrich would claim that "the average American just thinks this is a political statement" and "an aggressive act that is offensive,"[87] Bloomberg remarked that "we would be untrue to the best part of ourselves—and who we are as New Yorkers and Americans—if we said no to a mosque in Lower Manhattan."[88]

PRIORITIES AND POWER

Inevitably, as it did for the World Trade Center site, matters of power surrounded the controversy over 9/11. Ironically, however, none of the three most prominent voices surrounding the project—despite all their maneuverings—achieved their purported goals. The Islamic Community Center's Imam, Feisal Abdul Rauf, left the project after disputes with El-Gamal, the project's developer, and thereafter had to maintain his support for the project from the sidelines. Pamela Geller, perhaps the most vocal opponent of the "Ground Zero Mosque," succeeded in preventing a community center from being built, but now decries the fact that the site will contain an Islamic museum.[89] Finally, El-Gamal, the project's developer, eventually settled for building a vast apartment complex and a much scaled-down Islamic museum, recognizing that he will need to create his initial vision in a different location.[90] This all stands in contrast to the World Trade Center site, where, while ideas for what should be constructed differed dramatically, everyone agreed that *something* should be built. Park51 lacked any such fundamental consensus. Furthermore, the conflict surrounding Park51 illuminated one legacy of 9/11 with the growth of anti-Muslim ideologues seizing upon a local zoning question to kindle controversy far beyond the boundaries of Lower Manhattan.[91]

## Comparing the First Five Years after 9/11 and Park51

In the first year following 9/11, the *New York Times* focused on everyday New Yorkers' desire for things to return to normal. In particular, New Yorkers initially questioned whether their desire to move on and reconstruct their lives disrespected those who had died. During this period, entertainment venues, including movies, theaters, or sports arenas, were especially popular ways for New Yorkers to connect with one another. Over time, however, the abstract idea of returning to normal was eclipsed by more pragmatic concerns, such as the mechanics of actually rebuilding the World Trade Center site. At first, some victims' relatives were portrayed in the *New York Times* as public representatives and tangibly affected the rebuilding process, leading to a proliferation of new designs and pledges to honor the fallen. Nevertheless, our analysis of articles published in the *New York Times* suggested that attention to the public voice significantly waned over time. In the fourth and fifth years following 9/11, prominent designers and elected officials engaged in conflict over the fate of World Trade Center site, and such persons thus came to determine the future of Ground Zero.

The controversy over Park51 echoed these themes, as proponents and opponents of the Islamic community center fought over whether allowing this site to be built in Lower Manhattan somehow dishonored the dead, with the "Ground Zero Mosque" used as a spectacle for electioneering politicians and Islamophobic agitators to foment vitriolic opposition and insert themselves into national news coverage. The question of public voice also arose here, with community members and victims' relatives initially given space to express their approval or disapproval towards plans for the site. As in the first five years after 9/11, however, politicians, pundits, and inflammatory ideologues who appealed to the public interest but acted semiautonomously eventually eclipsed these voices. Nonetheless, as opposed to the World Trade Center site, where prominent voices at least agreed that something should be constructed, Park51 eventually fell victim to the incompatible interests surrounding it.

## Conclusion

Ultimately, we believe that this study provides (at least) three lessons for those interested in the nature and ramifications of large-scale disasters on those people and places most affected. First, and perhaps most important for future scholarship, is the recognition that the longer aftermath of a disaster is a multifaceted event and cannot simply be understood by viewing a single affected community, as many 9/11 studies have done; through short-term dynamics at a broad level; or through gathering the many individual traumas. Rather, as we have sought to do here, one must also understand the common priorities that emerge in a disaster's aftermath, and how these priorities are debated, contested, and shape everyday experiences and lived interactions. In other words, studies of disaster must focus on people at individual, group, and collective levels.

Second, we hope to have shown that newspaper articles, despite their limitations, offer a rich and unparalleled resource for those studying such everyday experiences and lived interactions. As the first draft of history, newspapers describe particulars of events and lives, offering detailed accounts of individual and civic challenges and responses that can be analyzed over time. Thus, the New York Times coverage of the five years after 9/11 and for the Park51 controversy allowed us to trace the post–9/11 trajectory as key issues emerged and underwent change, offering insight into how disasters can play out temporally.

At the same time, this methodological approach, guided by thematic coding that identified prominent topics in the news, may have missed topics that were also important and of concern to groups that are typically underrepresented in media discourse. For example, here we did not discuss the striking disparities in death compensation that disproportionally benefitted families with high rather than low-wage earners[92] and disbursements to some kinds of businesses over others,[93] issues that would have been situated in our "compensation" category. Our study's categorization therefore streamlined but also narrowed our focus, which we ultimately see as a both limitation and a contribution of our work: Rather than start with a priori categories that would have limited our exploration of the news, we used the news articles themselves to develop these categories.[94] Guided by frequency statistics, these categories then permitted us to trace the larger post–9/11 trajectory, and reveal details about how people, as individuals and groups, experienced New York City after this cataclysmic event.

Finally, this chapter both confirms and complicates Stanley Cohen's thesis that following a disaster, a community either "recovers its former equilibrium or achieves a stable adaptation to the changes which the disaster may have brought about."[95] As we have shown, immediately following 9/11, New Yorkers desperately sought to resume normality and regain a former equilibrium. At the same time, they feared doing so would disrespect the memory of those lost on 9/11. This tension emerged in the disparity between socioemotional and economic values as rebuilding the World Trade Center commenced, and reemerged once more in the Park51 controversy between those who felt that building an Islamic Community Center was disrespectful to the memory of the tragedy and those that felt such a project was an affirmation of core American values. Ironically, this resulted in the return of a sort of normality as somewhat familiar economic and political conflicts returned to dominate the public discourse.

As this study and the rest of the chapters in this book show, however, this new equilibrium provided a host of novel complications and uncertainties all of its own, concerning debates over American ideals and identity, the meaning of Islam,[96] and how to properly commemorate and respect a site of great horror. For example, Park51, as a "planned sign of tolerance,"[97] will not be constructed as a monument to New York City's cosmopolitanism and inclusionary ethos. As this vividly illustrates, although various factions attempted to influence the rebuilding of Lower Manhattan, at the forefront of this process was a combination of vested economic interests and debates over the role of those striving communities and individual stories that make up the tapestry of this vibrant city of immigrants.

# Appendix A

*Breakdown of Subcategories by Year*

*New York Times* Articles: "World Trade Center Rebirth"

| | 2001 | 2002 | 2003 | 2004 | 2005 | 2006 | Totals |
|---|---|---|---|---|---|---|---|
| **1 Professional/ architectural planning** | 20 | 50 | 54 | 30 | 12 | 10 | 176 |
| | R=11.36% | R=28.41% | R=30.68% | R=17.04% | R=6.81% | R=5.68% | R=99.98% |
| | C=15.27% | C=31.06% | C=42.86% | C=40.00% | C=20.00% | C=15.87% | C=28.57% |
| **2 Political issues** | 13 | 35 | 19 | 11 | 26 | 27 | 131 |
| | R=9.92% | R=26.72% | R=14.5% | R=8.40% | R=19.85% | R=20.61 | R=100% |
| | C=9.92% | C=21.74% | C=15.08% | C=14.67% | C=43.33% | C=42.86% | C=21.27% |
| **3 Business/ economic** | 40 | 18 | 8 | 9 | 6 | 13 | 94 |
| | R=42.55% | R=19.15% | R=8.51% | R=9.57% | R=6.38% | R=13.83% | R=99.99% |
| | C=30.53% | C=11.18% | C=6.35% | C=12.00% | C=10.00% | C=20.63% | C=15.26% |
| **4 Return to normal** | 43 | 18 | 11 | 6 | 2 | 2 | 82 |
| | R=52.44% | R=21.95% | R=13.41% | R=7.32% | R=2.44% | R=2.44% | R=100% |
| | C=32.82% | C=11.18% | C=8.73% | C=8.00% | C=3.33% | C=3.17% | C=13.31% |
| **5 Citizens' participation in planning** | 2 | 22 | 24 | 7 | 6 | 4 | 65 |
| | R=3.08% | R=33.85 | R=36.92 | R=10.77 | R=9.23% | R=6.15% | R=100% |
| | C=1.53% | C=13.66% | C=19.95% | C=9.33% | C=10.00% | C=6.35% | C=10.55% |

| | 1 | 2 | 3 | 4 | 5 | 6 | 7 |
|---|---|---|---|---|---|---|---|
| 6 Sadness/ melancholy | 5 R=15.15% C=3.82% | 7 R=21.21% C=4.35% | 5 R=15.15% C=3.97% | 8 R=24.24% C=10.67% | 4 R=12.12% C=6.67% | 4 R=12.12% C=6.35% | 33 R=99.99% C=5.36% |
| 7 Cleanup | 6 R=31.58% C=4.58% | 7 R=36.84% C=4.35% | 1 R=5.26% C=0.79% | 2 R=10.53% C=2.67% | 2 R=10.53% C=3.33% | 1 R=5.26% 1.59% | 19 R=100% C=3.08% |
| 8 Progress and deadlines | 2 R=12.5% C=1.57% | 4 R=25% C=2.48% | 4 R=25% C=3.17% | 2 R=12.5% C=2.67% | 2 R=12.5% C=3.33% | 2 R=12.5% C=3.17% | 16 R=100% C=2.60% |
| Totals | 131 R=21.27% C=100.04% | 161 R=26.14% C=100% | 126 R=20.45% C=100.09% | 75 R=12.18% C=100.01% | 60 R=9.74% C=99.99% | 63 R=10.23% C=99.99% | 616 |

## Notes

1. This chapter is not meant to provide any sort of exhaustive literature on the topic of "disaster." Rather, its purpose is to provide some background context for the sections that follow. For more extensive information on the topic of "disaster," see, e.g., Fischer, 1994; Gist, Lubin, and Redburn, 1999; Prince, 1920; Reyes, 2006; Stehr, 2006.
2. Thornburg, Knottnerus, and Webb, 2007.
3. Ibid.
4. Drabek and McEntire, 2003.
5. Dynes, DeMarchi, and Pelanda, 1987.
6. Fritz, 1961, 655.
7. Dynes, 1970.
8. Cohen, 1972.
9. Ibid., 23.
10. Erickson, 1994.
11. Ibid., 229; italics in the original.
12. Stellman et al., 2008.
13. 9/11 Commission, 2011.
14. See, for example, DiMarco, 2007; Foner, 2005; Greenberg, 2003; Linenthal, 2005.
15. See, for example, Boss, 2004; Carll, 2007; Coates, Rosenthal, and Schechter, 2003; Danieli, Dingman, and Zellner, 2005.
16. Amer and Bagasra, 2013; see also "Living in Houses without Walls: Muslim Youth in New York City in the Aftermath of 9/11" in this book.
17. See, for example, Northouse, NetLibrary Inc., and Computer Ethics Institute, 2006; Proske, 2008.
18. Ortiz, Myers, Walls, and Diaz, 2005; see also Downs, 1972.
19. McCarthy, McPhail, and Smith, 1996.
20. Earl, Martin, McCarthy, and Soule, 2004; Martin and Hansen, 1998; Salles, 2010.
21. With appreciation for the work of Jerry Fletcher, Sarah Gyorog, Vicki Myers, Lorraine Phillips, and Sarah Woodside.
22. See "Mirrored Reflections: (Re)Constructing Memory and Identity in Hiroshima and New York City" in this book; see also Low, Taplin, and Lamb, 2005; Low, 2004.
23. Kirk Johnson, "For a City Still in Shock, Picking up Life's Routine," *New York Times*, September 20, 2001.
24. Jesse McKinley, "New York's Theaters and Museums Open in a Bold Resolve to Persevere," *New York Times*, September 14, 2001.
25. Michelle O'Donnell, "Getting Back to Normal, Whatever That Is," *New York Times*, October 7, 2001.
26. Robin Pogrebin, "At 'Phantom,' Empty Seats and Defiance," *New York Times*, September 20, 2001.

27. Ibid.

28. Rick Lyman, "In Little Time, Pop Culture is Almost Back to Normal," *New York Times*, October 4, 2001.

29. Ibid.

30. Ben Ratliff, "Jazz Clubs Swing Back to Life," *New York Times*, October 19, 2001.

31. McKinley, "New York's Theaters and Museums Open."

32. Ibid.

33. Herbert Muschamp, "Ground Zero: 6 New Drawing Boards," *New York Times*, October 1, 2002.

34. David W. Dunlap, "Architects' Clashing Visions Threaten to Delay World Trade Center Tower," *New York Times*, October 23, 2003; David W. Dunlap, "After Year of Push and Pull, 2 Visions Meet at 1,776 Feet," *New York Times*, December 26, 2003.

35. Deutsch, 1982.

36. Ibid.

37. Edward Wyatt, "Six Plans for Ground Zero, All Seen as a Starting Point," *New York Times*, July 17, 2002.

38. Ibid.

39. Ibid.

40. Charles V. Bagli, "Trade Center Leaseholder Braces for Battle; Proposed Land Swap and Changed Developmental Plan Imperil Silverstein," *New York Times*, August 17, 2002.

41. Edward Wyatt, "7 Design Teams Offer New Ideas for Attack Site," *New York Times*, December 19, 2002.

42. Edward Wyatt, "Fewer Offices, More Options in Planning for Ground Zero," *New York Times*, October 10, 2002.

43. Ibid.

44. Wyatt, "Six Plans," 2002.

45. Johnson, "For a City," 2001.

46. Cf. Patrick D. Healy, "Leading Donors to Pataki PAC in 2004 Included Developers of Ground Zero," *New York Times*, January 22, 2005.

47. Patricia Cohen, "Laying Unidentified Remains to Rest," *New York Times*, June 4, 2012.

48. See, for example, Patrick D. Healy and Charles V. Bagli, "Pataki and Bloomberg Endorse Changes in Ground Zero Tower," *New York Times*, May 5, 2005.

49. Pogrebin, "At 'Phantom,' Empty Seats," 2001.

50. Healy and Bagli, "Pataki and Bloomberg Endorse," 2005.

51. Charles V. Bagli, "Disputes Over 9/11 Site Simmer on," *New York Times*, November 9, 2005.

52. Ibid.

53. For a more detailed analysis of the political struggles in the rebuilding of One World Trade Center, see Mollenkopf, 2005; Sagalyn, 2016.

54. Javier C. Hernandez, "Vote Endorses Muslim Center Near Ground Zero," *New York Times*, May 26, 2010.

55. Javier C. Hernandez, "Planned Sign of Tolerance Bringing Division Instead," *New York Times*, July 13, 2010.

56. Ibid.

57. Ibid.

58. Sweeney and Opotow, 2013.

59. Paul Vitello, "Imam Steps down from Project near Ground Zero," *New York Times*, February 4, 2011.

60. "Photo Exhibit at Park51," *New York Times*, August 8, 2011.

61. Matt Flegenheimer, "Islamic Center and Mosque Near Ground Zero Imperiled by Rent Dispute," *New York Times*, October 16, 2011.

62. Ronda Kaysen, "Condo Tower to Rise Where Muslim Community Center Was Proposed," *New York Times*, May 12, 2017.

63. Ibid.

64. Ibid.

65. Ralph Blumenthal and Sharaf Mowjood, "Muslim Prayers Fuel Spiritual Rebuilding Project by Ground Zero," *New York Times*, December 8, 2009.

66. Hernandez, "Vote Endorses Muslim Center."

67. Hernandez, "Planned Sign of Tolerance."

68. Clyde Haberman, "An Islamic Center, and What Belongs by Ground Zero," *New York Times*, May 27, 2010.

69. Ibid.

70. "Pamela Gellar: In Her Own Words," *New York Times*, October 8, 2010.

71. Damien Cave, "Far from Ground Zero, Obscure Pastor Is Ignored No Longer," *New York Times*, August 25, 2010.

72. Sweeney and Opotow, 2013.

73. Michael Barbaro, "Political Leaders' Rift Grows on Muslim Center," *New York Times*, August 25, 2010.

74. Anne Barnard and Alan Feuer, "Outraged, and Outrageous," *New York Times*, October 10, 2011.

75. Michael M. Grynbaum, "Islamic Center Ad Shows Limits of M.T.A. Powers," *New York Times*, August 11, 2010.

76. Michael Barbaro, "Jewish Group Opposes Muslim Center Near Ground Zero," *New York Times*, July 30, 2010.

77. Edna Aizenberg, "Muslims and the Apology Question," *New York Times*, September 20, 2010.

78. Barbaro, "Political Leaders' Rift Grows."

79. Paul Vitello, "Islamic Center near Ground Zero Has New Imam," *New York Times*, January 14, 2011.

80. Ibid.

81. Kaysen, "Condo Tower to Rise."

82. Michael Barbaro and Marjorie Connelly, "New Yorkers Divided over Islamic Center, Poll Finds," *New York Times*, September 2, 2010.

83. Michael Barbaro, "Debate Heats up about Mosque near Ground Zero," *New York Times*, July 30, 2010.

84. Hernández, "Planned Sign of Tolerance."

85. Colin Moynihan, "Ex-Firefighter Argues against Proposed Muslim Center," *New York Times*, March 15, 2011.

86. Sweeney and Opotow, 2013.

87. Barbaro, "Jewish Group Opposes Muslim Center."

88. Jim Dwyer, "The Impossible Mayor of the Possible," *New York Times*, August 18, 2013.

89. Kaysen, "Condo Tower to Rise."

90. Ibid.

91. Indeed, within New York City, a shocking 2013 report documented that since 2002, the New York Police Department had embarked on a covert domestic surveillance program monitoring American Muslims throughout the Northeast that violated individuals' civil rights and had devastating impact. See "Living in Houses without Walls: Muslim Youth in New York City in the Aftermath of 9/11" in this book, and Shamas and Arastu, 2013.

92. Amanda Ripley, "WTC Victims: What's a Life Worth?" *Time*, February 6, 2002.

93. Dixon and Stern, 2004.

94. This is consistent with the work of psychologist Klaus Holzkamp (1992), who critiqued empirical research as problematically narrowed by a priori categories.

95. Cohen, 1972.

96. See "Living in Houses without Walls: Muslim Youth in New York City in the Aftermath of 9/11" in this book.

97. Hernandez, "Planned Sign of Tolerance."

## References

9/11 Commission. *The 9/11 Commission Report: Final Report of the National Commission on Terrorist Attacks Upon the United States*. New York: Norton, 2011.

Amer, Mona M., and Anisah Bagasra. "Psychological Research with Muslim Americans in the Age of Islamophobia: Trends, Challenges, and Recommendations." *American Psychologist* 68, no. 3 (April 2013): 134–144.

Boss, Pauline. "The Burgess Award Lecture: Ambiguous Loss Research, Theory, and Practice: Reflections after 9/11." *Journal of Marriage and Family* 66, no. 3 (2004): 551–566.

Carll, Elizabeth K. *Trauma Psychology: Issues in Violence, Disaster, Health, and Illness*. Westport, CT: Praeger, 2007.

Coates, Susan W., Jane L. Rosenthal, and Daniel S. Schechter. *September 11: Trauma and Human Bonds*. Hillsdale, NJ: Analytic Press, 2003.

Cohen, Stanley. *Folk Devils and Moral Panics: The Creation of the Mods and Rockers*. London: MacGibbon and Kee Ltd, 1972.

Danieli, Yael, Robert L. Dingman, and Jennifer Zellner. *On the Ground after September 11: Mental Health Responses and Practical Knowledge Gained*. New York: Haworth Maltreatment and Trauma Press, 2005.

Deutsch, Morton. 1982. "Interdependence and Psychological Orientation." In *Cooperation and Helping Behavior: Theories and Research*, edited by Valerian Derlega and Janusz L. Grzelak, 16–41. New York: Academic Press, 2013.

DiMarco, Damon. *Tower Stories: An Oral History of 9/11*. Santa Monica, CA: Santa Monica Press, 2007.

Dixon, Lloyd, and Rachel Kaganoff Stern. *Compensation for Losses from the 9/11 Attacks*. Santa Monica, CA: Rand Corporation, 2004.

Downs, Anthony. "Up and down with Ecology-the Issue-Attention Cycle." *Public Interest* 28 (1972): 38–50.

Drabek, Thomas E., and David A. McEntire. "Emergent Phenomena and the Sociology of Disaster: Lessons, Trends and Opportunities From the Research Literature." *Disaster Prevention and Management: An International Journal* 12, no. 2 (2003): 97–112.

Dynes, Russell, R. *Organized Behavior in Disaster*. Lexington, MA: Health Lexington Books, 1970.

Dynes, Russell R., Bruna DeMarchi, and Carlo Pelanda. *Sociology of Disasters: Contribution of Sociology to Disaster Research*. Milan: Franco Angeli, 1987.

Earl, Jennifer, Andrew Martin, John D. McCarthy, and Sarah A. Soule. "The Use of Newspaper Data in the Study of Collective Action." *Annual Review of Sociology* 30 (2004): 65–80.

Erikson, Kai. *A New Species of Trouble: The Human Experience of Modern Disasters*. New York: Norton, 1994.

Fischer, Henry W. *Response to Disaster: Fact Versus Fiction & Its Perpetuation—The Sociology of Disaster*. Lanham, MD: University Press of America, 1994.

Foner, Nancy, ed. *Wounded City: The Social Impact of 9/11 on New York City*. New York: Russell Sage Foundation, 2005.

Fritz, Charles E. 1961. "Disasters." In *Contemporary Social Problems: An Introduction to the Sociology of Deviant Behavior and Social Disorganization*, edited by Robert King Merton and Robert A. Nisbe, 651–694. New York: Harcourt, Brace and World, 1961.

Fullilove, Mindy Thompson, Lourdes Hernandez-Cordero, and Jennifer Stevens Madoff. "Promoting Collective Recovery Through Organizational Mobilization: The Post–9/11 Disaster Relief Work of NYC Recovers." *Journal of Biosocial Science* 36, no. 4 (2004): 479–489.

Gist, Richard, Bernhard Lubin, and Bradley G. Redburn. "Psychosocial, Ecological and Community Perspectives on Disaster Response." In *Response to Disaster*, edited by Richard Gist and Bernhard Lubin, 1–20. Philadelphia: Brunner/Mazel, 1999.

Greenberg, Judith. *After 9/11: Trauma at Home*. Lincoln: University of Nebraska Press, 2003.

Holzkamp, Klaus. "On Doing Psychology Critically." *Theory & Psychology* 2, no. 2 (1992): 193–204.

Ikle, Fred C., and Harry V. Kincaid. *Social Aspects of Wartime Evacuation of*

*American Cities: National Academy of Sciences-National Research Council Disaster Study 4.* Washington, DC: National Academy of Sciences, 1956.

Kreps, Gary A., and Thomas E. Drabek. "Disasters Are Non-Routine Social Problems." *International Journal of Mass Emergencies and Disasters* 14 (1996): 129–153.

Linenthal, Edward T. 2005. "The Predicament of Aftermath: Oklahoma City and September 11." In *The Resilient City: How Modern Cities Recover From Disaster,* edited by Lawrence J. Vale and Thomas J. Campanella, 55–74. New York: Oxford University Press, 2005.

Low, Setha M. "The Memorialization of September 11: Dominant and Local Discourses on the Rebuilding of the World Trade Center Site." *American Ethnologist* 31, no. 3 (2004): 326–339.

Low, Setha M., Dana H. Taplin, and Mike Lamb. "Battery Park City: An Ethnographic Field Study of the Community Impact of 9/11." *Urban Affairs Review* 40, no. 5 (2005): 655–682.

Martin, Shannon E., and Kathleen A. Hansen. *Newspapers of Record in a Digital Age: From Hot Type to Hot Link.* Westport, CT: Praeger, 1998.

McCarthy, John D., Clark McPhail, and Jackie Smith. "Images of Protest: Dimensions of Selection Bias in Media Coverage of Washington Demonstrations, 1982 and 1991." *American Sociological Review* (1996): 478–499.

Mollenkopf, John. *Contentious City: The Politics of Recovery in New York City.* New York: Russel Sage Foundation, 2005.

Northouse, Clayton, NetLibrary Inc., and Computer Ethics Institute. *Protecting What Matters Technology, Security, and Liberty Since 9/11.* Washington, DC: Brookings Institution Press, 2006.

Ortiz, David, Daniel Myers, Eugene Walls, and Maria-Elena Diaz. "Where Do We Stand With Newspaper Data?" *Mobilization: An International Quarterly* 10, no. 3 (2005): 397–419.

Prince, Samuel Henry. "Catastrophe and Social Change, Based Upon a Sociological Study of the Halifax Disaster." Ph.D. thesis, Columbia University, 1920.

Proske, Dirk. *Catalogue of Risks: Natural, Technical, Social and Health Risks.* New York: Springer, 2008.

Reyes, Gilbert. "International Disaster Psychology: Purposes, Principles and Practices." In *Handbook of International Disaster Psychology,* edited by Gilbert Reyes and Gerard A. Jacobs, 1–13. Westport, CT: Praeger, 2006.

Sagalyn, Lynne B. *Power at Ground Zero: Politics, Money, and the Remaking of Lower Manhattan.* New York: Oxford University Press, 2016.

Salles, C. "Media Coverage of the Internet: An Acculturation Strategy for Press of Record?" *Innovation in Journalism* 7, no. 1 (2010): 3–14.

Shamas, Diala, and Nermeen Arastu. *Mapping Muslims: NYPD Spying and Its Impact on American Muslims.* New York: CLEAR, MACLC, AALDEF, 2013. https://goo.gl/jxyXcy.

Stehr, Steven. D. "The Political Economy of Urban Disaster Assistance." *Urban Affairs Review* 41, no. 4 (2006): 492–500.

Stellman, Jeanne Mager, et al. "Enduring Mental Health Morbidity and Social Function Impairment in World Trade Center Rescue, Recovery, and Cleanup Workers: The Psychological Dimension of an Environmental Health Disaster." *Environmental Health Perspectives* 116, no. 9 (2008): 1248–1253.

Sweeney, Patrick, and Susan Opotow. "'Why There?' Islamophobia, Environmental Conflict, and Justice at Ground Zero." *Social Justice Research* 26, no. 4 (December 1, 2013): 492–512.

Thornburg, P. Alex, J. David Knottnerus, and Gary R. Webb. "Disaster and Deritualization: A Re-interpretation of Findings From Early Disaster Research." *Social Science Journal* 44, no. 1 (2007): 161–166.

# Mirrored Reflections
## (Re)Constructing Memory and Identity in Hiroshima and New York City

### Hirofumi Minami and Brian R. Davis

T he premier screening of the movie *Hiroshima Ground Zero*, held in New York City in April 2007, was notable insofar as it was wholly uncontroversial. The film had grown out of a 1998 production of "The Atomic-Bomb Dome and the Disappeared Town," a project that had recaptured scenes of Hiroshima as it existed before the August 6, 1945, atomic bombing at the close of World War II. The producers, in an effort to boost the resonance of the film for a contemporary American audience, had juxtaposed the words "Ground Zero" with the original title as an explicit link to the September 11, 2001, attack in New York City. Despite the organizers' concerns that this move might prove problematic, as they were mindful of lingering political contestation over the legitimacy of the US role in dropping the A-bomb and even "Remember Pearl Harbor" sentiment, the movie was well received and followed by productive discussion.[1]

The addition of the phrase "Ground Zero" to that film's title might appear unremarkable. After all, the original meaning of the term *ground zero* is "the heart of nuclear explosion" and "the deepest level of destruction,"[2,3] certainly themes readily associated with Hiroshima on both sides of the Pacific. Yet allusions linking "Ground Zero" to the bombing of Hiroshima have met with a sense of resistance or uneasiness since at least 2002, when the first author (Minami) began his research on the recovery process in post–9/11 New York City from the standpoint of second-generation *hibakusha* (translated literally: those who are exposed to nuclear radiation) of Hiroshima. Thus, nearly two decades after the events of 9/11, there remains a strong sense, in conversations with New York, that comparisons between New York and Hiroshima are somehow inappropriate.

In New York City, "Ground Zero" has come to denote not the destruction and absence of some nameless place but rather the ruins of the Twin Towers of the World Trade Center, once an indelible fixture of the skyline that was invested with the city's identity prior to 9/11. If buildings function as symbols,[4] landmark towers work as a defining element in "the image of the city," providing meaning and emotional bonding for city dwellers and temporary visitors alike.[5] When this urban site became Ground Zero—and rebuilding efforts began—it became a place "defined and redefined by a tyranny of meaning"[6] where memories of New York City as it had been seemed irreconcilable with the new reality of After. It is in this sense that *rebuilding* does not just concern the reconstruction of a vacated physical space; rebuilding also signifies an urban planning process for creating "new symbolic meaning [that] could possibly account for the traumatic experience, the 'moral shock' that the attack [on 9/11] had been for society."[7]

Given these complex processes for making meaning, efforts to analyze how the years-long rebuilding effort at New York City's Ground Zero abetted the process of healing after 9/11 have and will continue to prove a challenge.

A solution we propose with this chapter is employing a "Psychoanalysis of Cities" framework[8] for understanding the reconstruction of post–9/11 New York City through comparisons with another Ground Zero embedded within a historical constellation of events spanning decades: post–8/6 Hiroshima. We begin from the premise that healing is not accomplished by the architectural completion of memorial spaces alone. Rather, healing can be more expansively conceptualized as a collective process of symbol formation.[9,10] Through this often-contested process, we argue, it becomes possible to express "the unspeakable"[11] dimensions of collective trauma. In comparing and contrasting the complex memorial (re)construction processes in New York City and Hiroshima in particular, we argue, it becomes possible to analyze the collective act of remembering in both cities and how they have rethought recovery and identity within their urban landscapes. Following brief histories of the development of New York City's and Hiroshima's memorial sites, we critically analyze a spectrum of social and historical dynamics evident in the long-term recovery processes of these cities. Through our Psychoanalysis of Cities lens, we propose that both cities have for years been struggling to overcome unconscious resistance to addressing the traumatic loss of urban habitation and identity.

## (Re)Constructing New York: Listening to the City

Hajer writes that "rebuilding Ground Zero was never going to be an easy planning process" given "the complexity both in the production of meaning as well as the dramaturgical dynamics of the process."[12] The multiple players and stakeholders in this process included first responders; families of the victims; residents of Lower Manhattan; policymakers; business sectors; and local, state and regional bureaucracies—each themselves representative of multiple voices seeking to be heard. A chief challenge for reconstruction was going to involve how to coordinate these disparate groups into a workable, unified whole.

Recognizing the shortcomings of individual-oriented approaches to counter traumatic experiences at such a massive level, Fullilove and Hernandez-Cordero described an action-oriented research approach for facilitating the rebuilding of communities in post–9/11 New York.[13] They focused their efforts on the notion of "collective recovery," a multi-level systemic process for "the recovery of a community from injuries to its internal organization and its connection to other groups."[14] Specifically, in 2002 they helped facilitate community mobilization and reconnection strategies to target multiple groups and social organizations such as schools, churches, non-profit organizations, and commercial and governmental enterprises through a community-based alliance, NYC Recovers. Their central thesis was that organizations "were integral to the myriad communities that comprise the regional ecosystem, had the ability to assess the needs of their constituents, and [were best positioned to] institute appropriate remedies."[15]

Through connection with the NYC Recovers initiative, the first author joined a large-scale town meeting comprising more than 4,000 people selected to "represent the rich geographic, racial and income diversity of the metropolitan region." This community outreach event, "Listening to the City: Remember and Rebuild," was held at the Jacob Javits Center in New York City on July 20, 2002. The meeting was organized as a project of the Civic Alliance to Rebuild Downtown New York, a broad-based coalition of nearly one hundred groups committed to devising strategies for the redevelopment of Lower Manhattan. The meeting was described as a watershed event for the question of "how to arrive at a widely shared plan for rebuilding" Ground Zero and was deemed a

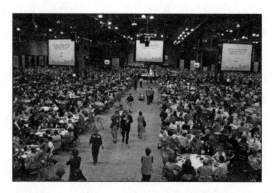

Figure 1. "Listening to the City: Remember and Rebuild" town meeting at the
Jacob Javits Center, New York City, July 20, 2002. Credit: LMDC

success "in terms of performing an open and transparent participatory
process."[16] We present this one-day meeting as ethnographic data derived
through the method of participant-observation, an approach entailing
first-person observation and collection of materials, interviewing, and
analysis of available newspaper articles and other archival data.[17]

During the interactive one-day session participants were grouped at
tables of ten to discuss pros and cons of six proposals for renewal of the
World Trade Center site. These original plans had been prepared in advance by the Lower Manhattan Development Corporation and the Port
Authority of New York and New Jersey. Proposal titles were thematic
permutations on *memorial*: "Memorial Plaza," "Memorial Square," "Memorial Triangle," "Memorial Garden," "Memorial Park," and "Memorial
Promenade." Proposed layouts varied in the number of towers (four to
six), street patterns, residential development, and the memorial space itself.
Facilitated small group discussions at each table were summarized on provided laptop computers and electronically compiled. Tallied results for
each question were displayed on large screens accompanied by commen-
tary text from select groups and individuals (Figure 1). These public sum-
maries were then fed back to the small groups for follow-up discussion.

This process was marked by a dynamic interplay among multiple
levels of agents. Discussions at each roundtable involved a back-and-
forth between individual participants' shared thoughts and feelings and
group discussion, with the goal of arriving at and submitting a consensus
opinion to the conveners. For their part, the conveners curated incoming
group feedback from the full forum, filtering their summary remarks fur-

ther through attention to the atmospheric reactions of the participating voices. It was a multimedia process as well, with ideas and feelings expressed in handwriting, on interactive laptop screens, and on large display screens, stimulating further reactions from attendees. The resulting composite opinions reflected a gradual accumulation of representative voices speaking for the mourning families, corporate interests, ethnic groups, community neighbors, religious minorities, and on behalf of all the citizens of New York City who were unable to attend.

Yet in Listening to the City, the organizers had opened a Pandora's box. Submitted messages began to take on a deeply emotional undercurrent of dissatisfaction with the proposed plans, as if to say, "none of them are good enough." At the end of this daylong session came a pivotal moment as the large screens proclaimed, "They're not New York"—a statement that seemed to resonate most powerfully with the audience. That moment marked the end to all six plans and their intricate and complex calculations of total office space, crossroad traffic, and open memorial space. The take-home message was clear: New York City is not just a big city. It has a special character as a dream city for innovation in art, business, and new ideas. The six bureaucratically approved plans for rebuilding Lower Manhattan, when carefully considered by four thousand representatives of the city, failed to embody the spirit of New York—of what it wants to be.

The unified voice of rejection at the Jacob Javits Center represented a turning point in the redevelopment process at Ground Zero.[18,19] As an alternate measure, the Lower Manhattan Development Corporation held an international design competition in December of 2002 that concluded with the selection of architect Daniel Libeskind as master planner of the World Trade Center site.[20] In Libeskind's speech for the proposal "Memory Foundations," the scene of his first encounter with the city was deployed to vivid effect:

> I arrived by ship to New York as a teenager, an immigrant, and like millions of others before me, my first sight was the Statue of Liberty and the amazing skyline of Manhattan. I have never forgotten that sight or what it stands for. This is what this project is all about.[21]

Libeskind's voice and story succeeded where the prior plans had failed, capturing the mythic sense of origin of arriving in the city and the meaning of the skyline as seen through the eyes of immigrants. He represented what New York City meant for those "millions of others before me." In epitomizing those who "arrived by ship to New York" with their myriad hopes and dreams, Libeskind succeeded in finding an overarching theme that encompassed different ethnicities, social classes, and political stances within a coherent vision of "what this project is all about."

However, much like the early promise of the Listening to the City event, this uplifting moment of shared vision was short-lived. Ongoing tensions between voices vying for representation were repeatedly pitted against a push for centralized control legitimized by economic and national policy. In the end, the execution of Libeskind's "Memory Foundations" met with years of complications resulting from delays, conflicts, revisions, and compromises in the redevelopment of the sixteen acres of the Ground Zero site.[22] Further complications accompanying the construction of the National September 11 Memorial and Museum from 2006–2014 essentially reproduced the basic conflict pattern set in the early years of redevelopment planning.

Our challenge in this chapter lies in trying to understand why it proved so difficult to find a redevelopment solution for post–9/11 Lower Manhattan that both honored the memories at Ground Zero and met the city's need for a particular collective identity. While practical difficulties concerning financing, resources, and planning were doubtless key factors in the lack of rapid resolution, the brief history we lay out here suggests that subtle psychological dynamics were also at work. The exercise in participatory democracy in the July 2002 Listening to the City event, as well as the delays in realizing Libeskind's subsequent vision, highlight the gradual and emotionally contentious formation of collective will to represent the identity of the city. Our need for a deeper understanding of the complex interaction of individual and group actors in the aftermath of 9/11 in New York City leads us to consider parallels with the decades-long memorial construction processes in Hiroshima after August 6, 1945.

## (Re)Constructing Hiroshima: Never to Repeat the Evil

A plain wristwatch, forever stopped at 8:15 on the morning of August 6, 1945, is one of the most well known exhibits at the Peace Memorial Museum at the center of the Peace Memorial Park in Hiroshima. The power of this artifact, often cited by popular media and academics alike, lies in its stark demarcation of Before and After, an encapsulation of the collective memory of the city and the birth of postwar Hiroshima's identity as a symbol of world peace. Yet potentially more illuminating for our present analysis are the series of complex social and financial negotiations behind the construction of Hiroshima's Peace Memorial Park.

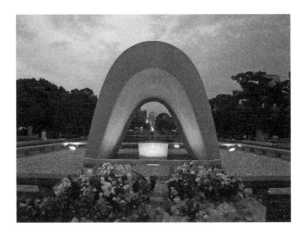

Figure 2. The cenotaph at the Peace Memorial Park in Hiroshima (taken by the first author on August 5, 2013). Written on the rectangular granite stone box is an epitaph that can be translated into English as "please rest in peace, for we shall not repeat the error." Credit: Hirofumi Minami

The task of coordinating the initial rebuilding effort fell to master planner Kenzo Tange, then a young associate professor at Tokyo University and modernist architect who integrated traditional components from ancient Japan and whose work was a prominent inspiration in the postwar period.[23] Tange's task was massive: construction of the Peace Center and Memorial Hall complex, a Convention Center, and a large Peace Memorial Park and its central memorial cenotaph, all fully integrated into overall city planning. The episode of the controversial planning, construction, and reception of the Peace Memorial cenotaph (Figure 2) exemplifies the representation dynamics at play—architecturally, politically, and psychologically—in Hiroshima's struggle to define a new postwar identity.

The cenotaph lay at the heart of Tange's Peace Memorial Park design and was originally assigned to sculptor Isamu Noguchi, another key planner of the Peace Memorial City. A *nisei* (second-generation Japanese born outside Japan) and American citizen, Noguchi had already earned the respect and support of both Tange and the mayor of Hiroshima by completing two approach bridges to the Peace Memorial Park.[24] In his submitted design for the central cenotaph, Noguchi envisioned the underground section as being a "place of solace to the bereaved—suggesting still further the womb of generations still unborn who would in time replace the dead."[25] At the same time, "the above ground was to be a symbol for all to see and remember."[26]

Despite high praise from master planner Tange and a proven track record with the approach bridges, Noguchi's original plan for the Peace Memorial Park cenotaph was ultimately rejected by the Hiroshima Peace Center and Park Committee just as construction was to begin. The rejection was driven mainly by the voice of one influential committee member and mentor to Tange, Hideto Kishida. Justifying his rejection, Kishida later wrote in his memoirs:

> It must be a wonderful thing that a Japanese architect and an American sculptor collaborate with each other to create a good work. But when it comes to the cenotaph at the center of the Hiroshima Peace Memorial Park, I'm not so sure. It is America that dropped the A-bomb, and we should not forget that Mr. Isamu Noguchi is an American.[27]

That Isamu Noguchi's stated artistic mission was of bridging East and West through a continual exploration of cultural identity only added a layer of irony to his being rejected because of his mixed heritage.[28] Forced to abandon Noguchi's original plan, Tange subsequently redesigned the cenotaph around an ancient Japanese roof form. The completed cenotaph was later unveiled in the summer of 1952, in time for the anniversary Peace Memorial Ceremony that August.

However, Tange's redesign opened a new chapter in the cenotaph controversy, this time regarding the Japanese wording of the stone epitaph at its center. The Hiroshima Peace Memorial Park cenotaph is distinctive in its anonymous character. A register of the names of the dead from the A-bombing is enclosed within a granite stone box under the roof;[29] no names of the dead are seen from outside. The official English translation of the brief epitaph, etched in Japanese on the front of the stone box, reads, "Let all the souls here rest in peace, for we shall not repeat the evil."[30] Read in the original Japanese, however, the second sentence lacks a grammatical subject. Together with the topic ayamachi wa ("the error" or "evil"), the conjugated verb kurikaeshimasenu ("not repeat") makes for a complete sentence as a subject-less vow.

The ambiguity of the absent subject of this epitaph—not naming who was in error—became the focal point in a decades-long series of disputes both locally and nationally. Summarizing the multitudinous and shifting interpretations as well as recurrent reactions over the epitaph, Ishida noted four distinct stages.[31] The chaotic initial reaction in the months following the opening of the cenotaph centered on accusations over the epitaph's repentant tone amidst emotional debates over Japan's responsibility for the war. Advocacy for US responsibility over dropping of the A-bomb by United Nations International Law Commission member and Indian jurist Radhabinod Pal in late 1952 served as a catalyst for further polarization that resulted in the solidification of two opposing positions. Anti-epitaph groups decried critical accusations that challenged their victim narrative of postwar Japan, while pro-epitaph groups appealed for Japan's role as peace-seeking agent. Heated controversy and, as we will argue, repressed emotions, were unleashed once more in 1957 with the publication of articles written by Memorial Park committee member Kishida. In them he openly criticized the epitaph as unsympathetic to "the many who died in the most cruel and unjust way."[32] Kishida's criticism of the epitaph succeeded mainly in stoking further mournful and open expressions of resentment for the A-bombing. After a period of relative stability, the 1969 government announced a repair plan for the by then aged cenotaph. This announcement reignited the dispute, this time over whether to preserve or change the epitaph, a debate that ended in 1970 on the side of preservation.[33]

## From One Ground Zero to Another: Collective Memories and Identities

Both the construction of war memorials and ritualistic performance of anniversaries serve as powerful cultural symbols of collective memory[34] and collective identity.[35] By collective memory we refer to a dynamic process of cultural knowledge that provides a shared medium of texts, images, and rituals within which a people can remember or articulate themselves as individuals and as members of a society.[36] Collective memory provides for "the localization of memories"[37]—for individuals as well as social groups such as families, cities, or nations—in order to render events comprehensible and therefore communicable. Cities in particular act as a "locus of collective memory" amidst associations of objects and places.[38] That is, cities help to stabilize and convey a society's self-image and identity, providing a shared cultural space for individuals to connect with and locate themselves within the shared symbols and stories of the society to which they belong.[39]

Paul Ricoeur has argued that history is about the past from the vantage of the present; history is analogous to the act of remembering as well as forgetting.[40] Collective memory is thus also a form of "re-presentation" for fashioning the past to the needs of the present.[41] However, this mal-leability of the past introduces an unavoidable tension between personal and collective memory in how they relate to and transform one another. Ricoeur provided an exposition of this tension through the bridging question, "Who remembers?"[42] That is, the pertinent question lies in *how* particular memory content (the *what* of memory) is ascribed to individual subjects or collectivities.

The problem of representation becomes particularly poignant when dealing with the traumas of August 6, 1945, and September 11, 2001. Crisis events can powerfully disrupt identity formation.[43] A sense of col-lective identity is suddenly cleaved from familiar and constitutive collec-tive memories as a city struggles to reinterpret itself after shared trauma. Collective efforts to reintegrate who we were in the past with what we are facing now and what we desire for our future become necessary during times of broken connections.[44] Commemorative practices thus serve as identity-building and meaning-making functions of collective memories, helping reconstruct, organize and reflect a crisis event into a shared—and sharable—experience.[45] Yet such practices cannot be accom-plished in isolation since what is at stake goes well beyond the individual to encompass material existence within a larger social framework—a hab-itable place, a *city*.

Against this theoretical backdrop, we view memorial architecture as "a key discursive space in which collective identities are reflected and maintained."[46] Our question is: how have practices of memory, identity and mourning been carried out in the actual events, dealings and debates marking the reconstruction planning processes in post–9/11 New York City and post–8/6 Hiroshima? For even if we agree upon the workings of collective memory and collective identity as key factors in understanding the rebuilding of these Ground Zeros, without further analysis it remains unclear how individual voices become "collective agency."[47] The task therefore remains for us to fill or bridge the gap between individual and collective levels of experiencing and acting in representing the trauma of these two cities.

## A Psychoanalysis of Cities Approach

Recovery of a missing place is a complex technical task, one that requires the reinstituting of meanings both sharable and grounded in the dynamic and multiple historical and psychological contexts of that particular place. To do justice in representing such multilayered contexts an interpretive action with respect to the forgotten or buried meanings of the site is needed.[48] Needed also is an analytic approach sensitive to the dynamic interplay of individual, interpersonal, and collective levels of a city as a life-world domain.[49]

Psychoanalysis of Cities is called upon here as an interpretive endeavor dealing with the collective, unconscious processes underlying construction and reconstruction of urban spaces. Psychoanalysis, here, is utilized as a general "theoretical perspective and [set of] technical rules for the interpretation of symbolic structures."[50] Within a Psychoanalysis of Cities approach, memorials are symbolic structures similar to dream images that are interpretable within a psychoanalytic framework. Memorials thus mediate individual and collective memories. Utilizing this approach, we next present our analysis of three overlapping themes relevant to both post–8/6 Hiroshima and post–9/11 New York City: representing the unspeakable, reflecting the mental images of historical agents, and working through repressed traumatic memories.

*Representing the Unspeakable*

Attempts at fashioning a new Great Story of collective identity can be halting and reopen old wounds as new aspects of the unspeakable slowly— sometimes over decades—are given voice. A typical storytelling of the A-bombing of Hiroshima starts on *that morning*, juxtaposing an idyllic setting against the horror that followed: "On August 6, 1945, the morning started with a cloudless blue sky characteristic of the Inland Sea's summer" abruptly riven by "the flash."[51] We do not with this description seek to minimize the experiences of individuals for whom such memories remain deeply personal. Yet we see another dimension in the collective memory of August 6, 1945 that is ascribed to the experience of Hiroshima as represented in master planner Tange's Peace Memorial City. Critically reviewing the collective memories of the A-bomb survivors of Hiroshima and Nagasaki during the postwar period, Okuda observed that within a span of ten years there developed a gradual collective identity of Japan as "the only A-bombed nation."[52] This observation is also consonant with a critical view of the dominant role played by nationalization policies in which a proliferation of narratives coded *Hiroshima* as the symbolic self-image of a victimized Japanese people and the nation's salvation in becoming a beacon of world peace.[53]

Yet the emphasis on the symbolism of *peace* during the postwar redevelopment of Hiroshima[54] appears paradoxical when we also consider the city's prior role not only as a commercial and academic hub but also as a major military center in the half-century leading up to and during World War II. Yet this uncomfortable past remained buried for decades. Indeed, nearly fifty years passed before the exhibition of A-bomb survivor experiences in the Peace Memorial Museum directly addressed the prewar period.[55] This latency period has marked a necessary interval for the city's and nation's initial response to the trauma of August 6, 1945.

And this response continues decades after the event. A district that remained virtually intact nearly forty years after the A-bombing was eventually cleared out from Hiroshima's landscape as part of an urban renewal project. The city's act of urban erasure, albeit unconsciously, served at least in part to cancel unwanted trace memories of a wounded past. The old image did not fit with the city's new identity as a hopeful place directed to the future.[56] Such instances of collective amnesia reveal the difficulty of representing a historical memory rendered unspeakable by traumatic events.

Are we also observing attempts at representing the unspeakable in post–9/11 New York City, of transforming the city's fractured self-image of invulnerability into a state of relative psychological equilibrium?[57] In contrast to the unified government response in Hiroshima, we see a plurality of voices reflective of the rich tapestry of ethnicities, languages, and cultures of New York City all clamoring for validation, often at odds, very publicly, with the regional and national bureaucracy. As the rebuilding of New York City's Ground Zero began in earnest in spring 2006, Gutman notes, the public, already frustrated by years of unfulfilled promises of urban renewal, were allowed for the first time to view the site for themselves.[58] Encountering only a "frozen material state"[59] still devoid of the tangible proof of reconstruction, the public began to dismiss the unrealistically optimistic official narratives in favor of their own "spaces and voices" through "appropriation and re-use of the site [that] countered the dominant and formal framing of the events."[60]

A "politics of memory"[61] aptly describes an emergent collective identity of Ground Zero as "a site where practices of memory and mourning have been in active tension with representational practice and debates over aesthetics."[62] Even the selection of Libeskind as master planner in rebuilding Lower Manhattan, a move coded by some as a "redemptive" attempt to provide a unified, representational vision, failed to stem the larger debate over the aesthetics of memory.[63] This debate is not likely to fade easily as the reconstruction process continues well into its second decade. The rebuilding of Ground Zero in New York City not only needs to address the architectural complexity of the task but also the psychological ramifications of the mourning process as the dark pits left in the streets and hearts of the city are gradually filled.

*Reflecting the Vorstellung of Historical Agents*

The absence of a subject in the epitaph at the heart of Hiroshima's Peace Memorial cenotaph provides a stark contrast to the 9/11 Memorial, where the names of those who are to be remembered comprise the main surface of the structure. The subjectless epitaph instead provides discursive space for questions of "who remembers"[64] and *who* takes action as a consequence of claiming responsibility for what happened. That is, as the subject is not prescribed, the act of representing becomes a symbolic and social action, with the actor subsequently positioned as historical agent. The place memory in this sense is not a mere summation of many individual memories but rather a dynamic production of a *Vorstellung*— Hegel's concept for "picture-thinking," or a mental image of a collective representation[65]—of the social collectivity at a time of crisis or loss. The designing and actual construction of memorials thus constitutes a form of symbolic reconstruction of place memories in the absence of the lost life-world.

The rejection of Isamu Noguchi's original design for the Hiroshima Peace Memorial City cenotaph is here interpreted as a collective reaction to the *nisei* artist's self-described attempts to transcend the nationalistic ideologies permeating the memorial project. Noguchi's stated goal of bridging East and West came across to his contemporaries rather as an egotistical rejection of the *Vorstellung* of those who were to be remembered. Kenzo Tange's final design, with its subject-less epitaph, was deemed a more fitting memorial for the tens of thousands of nameless Japanese dead.

In contrast to the closed bureaucratic process of the Hiroshima Peace Memorial planning, in retrospect what we saw at the Jacob Javits Center in New York City was democracy in practice. Despite a subsequently contested privileging of dominant voices,[66] the Listening to the City meeting largely fulfilled its title's promise in becoming an exercise in representation dynamics through a dialectically creative interplay of individual and collective levels of agency. It was a creative phenomenon in the sense it was wholly emergent—the collectivity did not exist prior to the appearance of a concrete body of expression. Through the presentation of ideas, pictures, and visions, four thousand previously undifferentiated participants at a public gathering were transformed into embodied agents positioned to lend or withhold support and approval. In the end, it was their unified voice that expressed the collective identity of the city rather than any of the six initial designs presented. That collective voice drew upon the mythical origins of New York City, and the nation, as founded and invigorated by immigrants. Evident in this shared sentiment are the multi-layered social frameworks that locate individual identities and memories of those who attribute "New York-ness" to their shared place identity.[67]

The recurrent struggles and subsequent conflicts surrounding the re-building of these two Ground Zero memorial sites propelled a gradual reshaping of their respective social frameworks. From the interpretive perspective afforded by a Psychoanalysis of Cities approach, this reshaping reflects efforts to construct a new collective identity capable of encompassing both the actual physical state of the city as well as the meaning structures of the life-world. Such meanings are in turn linguistically organized and culturally transmitted,[68] an ongoing process constituting the historical continuity of a place.

### Working Through Suppressed Memories

We have thus far argued for the gradual formation of cities as social frameworks reflecting a process for "the localization of memories"[69] through symbolically meaningful themes, such as may be found through architectural expression. Yet while symbols function as a consolidating nexus for collective identity, they often do so at the cost of losing diversity in the early stages of crisis. As a consequence, Bar-On reminds us, normalized discourses for dealing with the trauma of "the indescribable and the undiscussable" can have the unintended effect of helping "all parties avoid acknowledging the psychologically and morally painful parts of their respective biographies."[70]

Thus, efforts to represent layers of repressed memories too unspeakable to confront in the early phase of recovery—that is, "working through" the trauma[71]—are by necessity contested. Latency in recalling past memory is in turn understood as, ideally, an adaptive psychological mechanism for collective efforts to deal with the otherwise overwhelming task of physically and emotionally reconstructing the weakened agency of the city as a collective organization. At worst, however, avoidance of such acknowledgment can leave little recourse beyond triage as the full pain of the lost place identity erupts during periodic moments of social crisis.

In this latter scenario, the suppression of traumatic memory ensures that recovery efforts remain stymied by the unaddressed and unabated hemorrhaging of collective identity just under the city's surface. The dynamic relationship between collective memory and issues of identity that emerge in the struggle over representation constitutes what the memorial stands for, as well as for whom, at any given time.

Utilizing this analytic lens, we argue that the purpose achieved by the original symbolic deployment of peace as an overarching ideology for the reconstruction of post–8/6 Hiroshima was twofold: a vision for working through the overwhelming task of rebuilding the city amidst the postwar chaos and a desire to distance from an inconvenient militaristic past. Hiroshima's role as Peace Memorial City, epitomized in the subjectless epitaph, succeeded as a normalizing discourse of a new postwar identity[72]—yet the city gained this new identity at the cost of losing its past. Situational and external pressure during the postwar period, exerted by the US-led occupation and its strict regulation of the press code, contributed to the systematic suppression of views openly critical of the US role in dropping the A-bomb. Under such restrictive conditions, necessary to maintain the public image of peace, collective memory and identity became an outlet for the gradual releasing of raw emotions. In considering the controversy surrounding the Peace Memorial Park cenotaph, it is noteworthy that twelve years after the A-bombing these negative emotions were even more openly expressed than in the initial phase. Ishida attributed this latency to the overly idealistic notion inherent in the subject-less epitaph that placed the burden for unresolved emotions with the survivors,[73] with suppressed feelings sublimated into periodic disputes over the locus of ultimate responsibility—that is, the question of *who erred?*

The early phases of recovery in New York City, marked by a collective solidarity around an immigrant experience representative of what the city stands for, were gradually co-opted by the symbolic deployment of an aggressive "America first" jingoism, manifest in recent years most prominently by a powerful, vocally anti-immigrant nationalistic political movement.[74] The massive social forces forming the proactive and supportive ground for Libeskind's original "Memory Foundation" plan subsequently devolved into regressive bickering when the actual reconstruction process began.[75] Representation dynamics were dominated by politically partisan narratives and special interest sectors constituting Lower Manhattan, resulting in delays, conflicts, revisions, and mutually unsatisfying compromises.[76] By this stage of redevelopment, Ground Zero served more as a battlefield for political and commercial stakeholders as abstract figures of square feet, dollars, and traffic amounts once more took center stage within public debates. Yet this continual emergence and shifting of agents and issues also provides evidence that the process of working through is already underway in New York City. Taking the form of conflict rather than solution, the process of psychosocial recovery reflects an ongoing and emotionally vested struggle for a more inclusive image and place identity for the city.

## Lessons Learned: From Analysis to Healing

Both the Hiroshima Peace Memorial Park and the 9/11 Memorial in New York City were designed to provide a means of expressing the unsayable, to provide solace against an overwhelming collective trauma. Yet in doing so, a society's fixation on tangible monuments can also provide distancing and defensive strategies that "deflect the mourning process outwards and do not provide a living connection with the embodied side of experience, whether as a part of one's own history or as a result of transgenerational transmission."[77] Have the public narratives of healing in these two cities been reduced to their respective original symbolic visions for the reclamation of urban space at the cost of losing past identity? While we do not presume to advance an answer to this important question here, we cannot abrogate our shared responsibility to recognize and document the depth and longevity of both individual and collective psychological traumas visited upon these two Ground Zeros.

The interpretive works of several cultural theorists in recent years together paint a picture of the city of Hiroshima, restricted by decades after the war by an overly idealistic symbolism of peace, as a site of increasing collective efforts to resist repression of the original scene of Ground Zero.[78] Yet after more than seventy years, a full reckoning with the buried memories of a time up to August 6, 1945, may well be at hand. A multiplicity of voices and personalized narratives are slowly being recognized as the "missed traces of traumatic experiences" long displaced by official narratives of peace and nuclear nonproliferation.[79] In any event, such a long latency provides telling evidence of the depth of this city's pain, of the extent to which Hiroshima as collective subject has struggled to deal with its own memory and identity.

Measured against the more than half century marking the aftermath of Hiroshima post–8/6, the story of post–9/11 New York City's working through is still in its early chapters. Drawing upon the former case, we can conclude that attempts to overcome suppression of the original traumatic event might proceed in one of two directions. A sole focus on pragmatic solutions grounded in economic rationality, while promising near-term solutions, may lead to premature emotional closure as the original trauma is further rendered unspeakable. The alternative approach of further working through is the more difficult path, requiring the opening of ever deeper historical layers of the city's memory and identity. At present, we cannot tell which course New York City might take, but we are certain that in either eventuality as yet unresolved memories will burst forth repeatedly within the urban landscape for generations of city dwellers to come.

## Toward an Understanding of the Collective Healing Process

When researchers are faced with collective wounds at a massive scale— physical, emotional, metaphorical—they necessarily deal with resistance from both inner and outer domains. *Ground Zero* has come to embody in the collective imagination a tacit understanding of and symbolic meanings for the place and events of September 11, 2001. Reference to another Ground Zero—Hiroshima after its A-bombing on August 6, 1945—is missing in the current debates concerning the rebuilding of Lower Manhattan in New York City. The first author's own visceral sense of resistance to associating the phrase *Ground Zero*—now synonymous with 9/11—with the atomic bombing of Hiroshima provides a clue for the present investigation. Psychological resistance may indicate the working of largely unconscious feelings and reactions.[80] In the context of tensions and controversies surrounding the trauma preceding and during rebuilding of both Ground Zero sites, we can observe how such unconscious processes function at the level of collective memory and identity.

The notion of trauma as repressed memory, first pioneered by Freud and Breuer in their original formulation of hysteria, provided the foundation for subsequent studies on the long-term effects of aversive events at a massive scale.[81] Hysteric subjects, they wrote, "suffer for the most part from reminiscences": "The precipitating event in some way still continues to exercise an effect years later, not indirectly through a chain of intermediary causal links, but as a directly releasing cause, in something like the same way that a psychical pain remembered in waking consciousness will still produce the secretion of tears later on."[82]

Devastating events surpass the experiencer's psychological capacity, leaving no recourse other than to mentally block and dissociate from the shocking scenes through a process of "psychic numbing."[83] Such psycho-

logical defenses may take the form, in Japanese culture, of a mental "prohibition of don't look."[84] These defensive, unconscious processes take on
collective significance in the face of shared trauma: the experiencer is the
collective agency of an entire city. Yet such protective disconnection from
the event often produces unwanted consequences as pathological symptoms enter the experiencer's consciousness through a continual barrage of
repressed memories. Therapeutic interventions in the face of trauma lie in
efforts to retrieve the precipitating event in a less restrictive and defensive
way to enable the experiencer-as-agent to confront the full dimensions
of the original trauma. Healing thus constitutes a process for gradually
overcoming the suffering brought on by "reminiscences."

## Policy Implications

Hiroshima's international role as Peace Commemorative City has for decades publicly embodied the ideal of what former US President Barack
Obama described in May 2016 as "a future in which Hiroshima ... [is]
known not as the dawn of atomic warfare but as the start of our own
moral awakening."[85] Yet it is precisely the selected symbolism of peace
that has determined Hiroshima's place in contemporary world history,
predicated on an unconsciously "chosen trauma" of nuclear holocaust
and reinforced through multigenerational transmission.[86] Functional and
practical, the symbolism of peace defined a monolithic character for the
city, epitomized by Kenzo Tange's selection in designing the cenotaph
while rejecting contributions by diaspora artist Isamu Noguchi. Over seventy years after the event, both the military past of this city and the anger
of the *hibakusha* remain delicate topics under the idealistic public social
framing of the city. As long as the anger of the survivors of Hiroshima and
the memories of postwar nationwide resentment over the US attack and
occupation are repressed, human emotions will continue to burst forth
from unspeakable experience.

   As we have argued in this chapter, feelings of uneasiness encountered
in linking Hiroshima to Ground Zero in the context of New York City
touch upon largely unconscious processes of memory and identity common to survivors of 9/11. Political expediency and a human need for
emotional closure, in New York City and the nation alike, have and will
continue to give rise to optimistic narratives of renewal and recovery. The
voices of first responders, the families of 9/11 victims, and survivors alike
were gradually silenced to produce and preserve this national narrative.[87]
Consequently, as long as survivors' shared experiences are marginalized

through their framing as personal interest stories, the depth of those experiences, and pain, will remain untouched.

## Conclusions and Commitments

Our task with the present chapter has been to investigate the psychosocial processes underlying the formation of symbolic representations in the form of memorial building and reconstruction of two Ground Zero sites distant in time, Hiroshima and New York City. With our title, "mirrored reflections," we have attempted to provide a common psychoanalytic framework for considering the traumas visited upon these two cities. In doing so, our aim has been to analyze the collective acts of remembering and identification in how both cities have rethought recovery within their urban landscapes. Our reflections, of course, are not exhaustive and are limited by the scope of our individual life circumstances. Yet we argue that it cannot be otherwise, for there is no ground for psychoanalytic investigation other than starting from one's personal involvements. Further analysis of both apparent and latent symbolic structures and meanings as well as an interrogation of the mutually constitutive relationships between experiencer and memorial symbols is thus needed.

The wounds of both Ground Zeros remain vivid and aching, not only for the survivors themselves, but also for those of us who try to excavate the affected parts as academic researchers. In his pioneering work on survivors of Hiroshima, Robert Jay Lifton observed such psychodynamic processes in his attempt to listen to voices of *hibakusha* seventeen years after the event.[88] We join the survivors of both Ground Zeros in humility and gratitude as we share the painful process of overcoming resistance in the hope we may uncover layers of human consciousness overwhelmed by the unspeakable breakdown of the life-world after 8/6 and 9/11.

What lessons can be gleaned from post–8/6 Hiroshima to inform our understanding of the healing process after 9/11? The shared sense among the Javits Center attendees of New York City as a place deserving of a proper tribute to its unique character became apparent after the rejection of generic redevelopment proposals. Yet a dialectical tension between individual and collective agency in representing Ground Zero have both propelled and stymied the recovery. Hiroshima teaches us that the process of coming to terms with and comprehending the significance of 9/11 will continue to be difficult and slow. Any pronouncements on the realization of recovery will inevitably be subject to further interpretation of the experiences coming out of Ground Zero.

And so the question "Who remembers?" must remain an open one. We cannot know who stands before Hiroshima's Peace Memorial Park cenotaph or New York City's 9/11 Memorial reflecting pools, or what meanings each person takes away. Yet we argue that it is through these contemplative actions that we become historical agents capable of fashioning, reinterpreting, and enriching collective memories and identities. In reflecting on the relationship between these two Ground Zeros, we may also glimpse ways of giving voice to this liberating historical agency and for rebuilding our way to a better future.

## Notes

Both authors wish to express our deepest appreciation to Susan Opotow and Zachary Shemtob for their continuous support and editorial critiques as this chapter took shape, as well as to David Chapin of the Graduate Center, City University of New York, for his insightful comments and suggestions. The first author also wishes to express heartfelt thanks to Roger Hart of the Graduate Center, City University of New York for his support during fieldwork in New York. Gratitude also goes to the following organizations for supporting research activities conducted in New York and Hiroshima on which this chapter is based: the Department of Psychology of Hiroshima University; the Faculty of Human-Environment Studies of Kyushu University; the Graduate Center, City University of New York; Japanese Ministry of Education (MEXT) Fellowship Program for Japanese Scholars and Researchers to Study Abroad (2002); Japanese Grants-in-Aid for Scientific Research (Grant C. No. 21530658, 2009–11; Grant A. No. 23242056, 2011–15); and the Fulbright Fellowship Program for Foreign Researchers (2012–13).

1. Tanabe, 2008.
2. Sturken, 2004.
3. Gutman, 2009.
4. Whitehead, 1985.
5. Lynch, 1960.
6. Sturken, 2004.
7. Hajer, 2005, 445.
8. Minami, 2015.
9. Werner and Kaplan, 1984.
10. Zolberg, 1998.
11. Tanabe, 2008.
12. Hajer, 2005, 461.
13. Fullilove and Hernández-Cordero, 2006.
14. *Ibid.,* 160.
15. Fullilove and Saul, 2006, 171.

16. Hajer, 2005, 457.

17. Sato, 2006. An ethnographic approach usually entails a longer period of participant-observation, exemplified by previous fieldwork undertaken by the first author in Hiroshima. Participation by the first author in the Listening to the City meeting was complemented by continuous involvement with NYC Recovers activities, through which the author gained intersubjective validation of descriptions and interpretations of the acquired field data. Given these limitations, the historical reviews we present here should not be construed as being comprehensive but rather illustrative of a Psychoanalysis of Cities approach. Minami, 2015.

18. Nobel, 2005.

19. Hankin, 2012.

20. Sturken, 2004.

21. Cited in Hajer, 2005, 459.

22. Hankin, *2012*.

23. Fujimori, 2013.

24. Noguchi, 1968, 163. In Noguchi's own words, "The bridge with the rising sun was named *Tsukuru* ('to build') denoting life. The other bridge like a boat was *Yuku* ('to depart'). Having built, we die (through holocaust?)." The complex and even conflicting motivations evident in these words offer a glimpse into the complex act of building amidst a field of mass death.

25. Ibid., 164.

26. *Ibid.*

27. Kishida, 1958, 85.

28. Ashton, 1992.

29. Okuda, 2010.

30. Both the original verse and this English translation were prepared by Tadayoshi Saika, professor of English literature at Hiroshima University, at the request of the mayor of Hiroshima. Professor Saika used "we" deliberately to render the sentence more grammatically complete in English as well as retain the generalized subject of the act.Yoneyama, 1999, 24.

31. Ishida, 1997.

32. Kishida, 1958, 87.

33. That the public response to President Obama's 2016 visit to the Hiroshima Peace Memorial on the seventy-first anniversary of the atomic bombing excluded any mention of the epitaph is notable in this context insofar as the cenotaph controversy of the twentieth century has apparently receded in relevance.

34. Halbwachs, 1992; Connerton, 1989; Bal, Crewe, and Spitzer, 1999; Huyssen, 2003.

35. Baumeister, 1986; Pennebaker and Banasik, 1997.

36. Assmann and Czaplicka, 1995; Halbwachs, 1992, 52.

37. *Ibid.*

38. Rossi, 2002.
39. Kalinowska, 2012.
40. Ricoeur, 2004.
41. Halbwachs, 1992, 52; Ricoeur, 2004, 126.
42. *Ibid.*
43. Erikson, 1964.
44. Lifton, 1983.
45. Assmann and Czaplicka, 1995.
46. Jones, 2006. 564.
47. Bal, Crewe, and Spitzer, 1999, vii.
48. Boyer, 2001, 28; Low, 2004. In the latter article, Low draws on ethnographic data to document the suppressive role played by dominant discourses favoring a consumption-oriented approach to the memorialization process in the years immediately following 9/11. Her conclusions further highlight the necessity for understanding the underlying psychological processes leading to such domination at a collective level.
49. Habermas, 1987.
50. Habermas, 1971, 214; Habermas, 2001.
51. Japanese Broadcasting Corporation, 1977. The text of US President Barack Obama's speech during his May 27, 2016, official state visit to Hiroshima, the first for a sitting president since World War II, was nearly identical in its opening wording: "on a bright cloudless morning, death fell from the sky and the world was changed. A flash of light and a wall of fire destroyed a city." "Text of President Obama's Speech in Hiroshima, Japan," *New York Times*, May 27, 2016.
52. See also Okuda, 2010, 362.
53. Yoneyama, 1999, 24.
54. Ishimaru, 1988.
55. Okuda, 2010, 362.
56. Minami, 1997.
57. Jameson, 1982. We note, however, that "psychological equilibrium" may be a privilege afforded to some citizens over (or at the expense of) others. Critical social theory suggests that the silencing of certain voices within social spaces may in part be attributed to a "political unconscious" favoring dominant ideological narratives of social identity.
58. Gutman, 2009, 67.
59. *Ibid.*
60. *Ibid,.*
61. Huyssen, 2003.
62. Sturken, 2004, 312.
63. *Ibid.*, 321.
64. Ricoeur, 2004, 126.
65. Jameson, 2010, 21; Stace, 1955, 486.

66. Low, 2004.
67. Proshansky, Fabian, and Kaminoff, 1983.
68. Habermas, 1987.
69. Halbwachs, 1992, 52.
70. Bar-On, 1999, 4.
71. Freud, 1958.
72. The notion of a *"peace commemorating city"* also served important practical functions, both financial and political. First, this title distinguished Hiroshima from other war-inflicted cities as a means for the national government to justify its larger allocation of reconstruction funds. Second, the appellation complied with the directives of the US-led General Headquarters, Supreme Commander for the Allied Powers (GHQ/SCAP). Aware of public perceptions during the postwar occupation, GHQ/SCAP required a sensitive approach for dealing with a social landscape rife with potential anger within the nation generally and among the Hiroshima survivors in particular.
73. Ishida, 1997.
74. Gutman, 2009.
75. Hajer, 2005.
76. Nobel, 2005.
77. Kalinowska, 2012.
78. For example, see Naono, 2015. See also Okuda, 2010, 362; Yoneyama, 1999.
79. Naono, 2015, 181.
80. Freud, 1958.
81. See, for example, Herman, 1992.
82. Freud and Breuer, 2004) 11.
83. Lifton, 1967, 14.
84. Kitayama, 2010.
85. *"Text of President Obama's Speech in Hiroshima, Japan."* It is worthwhile here to highlight the handshake and conversation shared between Mr. Obama and ninety-one-year-old Sunao Tsuboi, chair of the Japan Confederation of A- and H-Bomb Sufferers Organizations, received wide coverage in the Japanese media. Played repeatedly, this wordless scene quickly became symbolic of a future-oriented reconciliation between the two countries despite a lack of admission (or accusation) of fault.
86. Volkan, 1998.
87. Gutman, 2009.
88. Lifton, 1967.

**References**

Ashton, Dore. *Noguchi: East and West.* Berkeley: University of California Press, 1992.
Assmann, Jan, and John Czaplicka. "Collective Memory and Cultural Identity."
    *New German Critique* 65 (1995): 125.

Bal, Mieke, Jonathan Crewe, and Leo Spitzer. *Acts of Memory: Cultural Recall in the Present.* Hanover, NH: University Press of New England, 1999.

Bar-On, Daniel. *The Indescribable and the Undiscussable: Reconstructing Human Discourse After Trauma.* Budapest: Central European University Press, 1999.

Baumeister, Roy F. *Identity: Cultural Change and the Struggle for the Self.* New York: Oxford University Press, 1986.

Boyer, M. Christine. *The City of Collective Memory: Its Historical Imagery and Architectural Entertainments.* Cambridge: Cambridge University Press, 2001.

Connerton, Paul. *How Societies Remember.* Cambridge: Cambridge University Press, 1989.

Erikson, Erik H. *Insight and Responsibility.* New York: Norton, 1964.

———. "Notes on Trauma and Community." In *Trauma: Explorations in Memory,* edited by Cathy Caruth, 183–199. Baltimore, MD: Johns Hopkins University Press, 1995.

Freud, Sigmund. "Remembering, Repeating and Working-Through (Further Recommendations on the Technique of Psycho-Analysis II)." In *The Standard Edition of the Complete Psychological Works of Sigmund Freud, Vol. 12,* edited by James Strachey and Anna Freud, 145–156. London: Hogarth Press and the Institute of Psycho-Analysis, 1958.

Freud, Sigmund, and Josef Breuer. *Studies in Hysteria.* Translated by N. Luckhurst. London: Penguin Books, 2004.

Fujimori, T. "The Importance of Kenzo Tange in the World." In *Kenzo Tange: Tradition and Creation,* edited by F. Kitagawa, 106–107. Tokyo: Bijutsu-Shuppansha, 2013.

Fullilove, Mindy T., and Lourdes Hernández-Cordero. "What Is Collective Recovery?" In *9/11: Mental Health in the Wake of Terrorist Attacks,* edited by Yuval Neria, Raz Gross, and Randall D. Marshall, 157–165. Cambridge: Cambridge University Press, 2006.

Fullilove, Mindy T., and Jack Saul. "Rebuilding Communities Post-Disaster in New York." In *9/11: Mental Health in the Wake of Terrorist Attacks,* edited by Yuval Neria, Raz Gross, and Randall D. Marshall, 166–177. Cambridge: Cambridge University Press, 2006.

Gutman, Yifat. "Where Do We Go from Here: The Pasts, Presents and Futures of Ground Zero." *Memory Studies* 2, no. 1 (2009): 55–70.

Habermas, Jurgen. *Knowledge and Human Interests.* Boston: Beacon Press, 1971.

———. *Theory of Communicative Action Volume Two: Life-World and System: A Critique of Functionalist Reason.* Translated by T. A. McCarthy. Boston: Beacon Press, 1987.

———. *The Liberating Power of Symbols.* Cambridge, MA: MIT Press, 2001.

Hajer, Maarten A. "Rebuilding Ground Zero: The Politics of Performance." *Planning Theory & Practice* 6, no. 4 (2005): 445–464.

Halbwachs, Maurice. *On Collective Memory.* Chicago: University of Chicago Press, 1992.

Hamai, S. *A-Bomb Mayor*. Hiroshima: Shift Project, 2011.

Hankin, Richard. *16 Acres: The Struggle to Rebuild Ground Zero*. DVD, Tanexis Productions, 2012.

Herman, Judith L. *Trauma and Recovery: The Aftermath of Violence—From Domestic Abuse to Political Terror*. New York: Basic Books, 1992.

Huyssen, Andreas. *Present Pasts: Urban Palimpsests and the Politics of Memory*. Stanford, CA: Stanford University Press, 2003.

Ishida, Y. "For to Repeat Faults We Shall Cease: Steps in the Epitaph Disputes." *Hiroshima Municipal Archives Bulletin* 20 (1997): 39–59.

Ishimaru, N. "The Process of Enactment of the 'Bill for Construction of Hiroshima: Eternal Peace Commemorative City' and Its Characteristics." *Hiroshima Municipal Archives Bulletin* 11 (1988): 1–56.

Jameson, Fredric. *Political Unconscious: Narrative as a Socially Symbolic Act*. Ithaca, NY: Cornell University Press, 1982.

———. *The Hegel Variations: On the Phenomenology of Spirit*. New York: Verso, 2010.

Japanese Broadcasting Corporation. *Unforgettable Fire: Pictures Drawn by Atomic Bomb Survivors*. New York: Pantheon Books, 1977.

Jones, Paul R. "The Sociology of Architecture and the Politics of Building: The Discursive Construction of Ground Zero." *Sociology* 40, no. 3 (2006): 549–565.

Kalinowska, Malgorzata. "Monuments of Memory: Defensive Mechanisms of the Collective Psyche and Their Manifestation in the Memorialization Process." *Journal of Analytic Psychology* 57 (2012): 425–444.

Kishida, Hideto. *En (Personal Encounters)*. Tokyo: Sagamishobou Publishing, 1958.

Kitayama, Osamu. *Prohibition of Don't Look: Living Through Psychoanalysis and Culture in Japan*. Tokyo: Iwasaki Gakujutsu Shuppansha, 2010.

Lifton, Robert J. *Death in Life: Survivors of Hiroshima*. New York: Random House, 1967.

———. *The Broken Connection: On Death and Continuity of Life*. Washington, DC: American Psychiatric Press, 1983.

Low, Setha M. "The Memorialization of September 11: Dominant and Local Discourses on the Rebuilding of the World Trade Center Site. *American Ethnologist* 31, no. 3 (2004): 326–339.

Lynch, Kevin. *The Image of the City*. Cambridge, MA: MIT Press, 1960.

Minami, Hirofumi. "Urban Renewal and the Elderly: An Ethnographic Approach." In *Handbook of Japan-United States Environment-Behavior Research: Toward a Transactional Approach*, edited by Seymour Wapner, Jack Demick, Takiji Yamamoto, and Takashi Takahashi, 133–148. New York: Springer, 1997.

———. "Toshino Seishin Bunseki (Psychoanalysis of Cities)." In *Workshops for Understanding Cities*, edited by Urban Design Course of Kyushu University, 16–23. Fukuoka: Kyushu University Press, 2015.

Naono, A. *Genbaku Taiken to Sengo Nippon (A-Bomb Experiences and Post-War Japan: Formation and Succession of Memories)*. Tokyo: Iwanami Publishing Company, 2015.

Neria, Yuval, Raz Gross, and Randall Marshall. *9/11: Mental Health in the Wake of Terrorist Attacks.* Cambridge: Cambridge University Press, 2006.

Nobel, Philip. *Sixteen Acres: Architecture and the Outrageous Struggle for the Future of Ground Zero.* New York: Henry Holt and Company, 2005.

Noguchi, Isamu. *A Sculptor's World.* New York: Harper & Row, 1968.

Okuda, Hiroko. *Genbaku no Kioku: Hiroshima Nagasaki no Shiso (Memories of the Atomic Bombing: Thoughts on Hiroshima and Nagasaki).* Tokyo: Keio Gijuku Daigaku Shuppankai, 2010.

———. "Remembering the Atomic Bombing of Hiroshima and Nagasaki: Collective Memory of Post-War Japan." *Acta Orientalia Vilnensia* 12, no. 1 (2011): 11–28.

Pennebaker, James W., and Becky L. Banasik. "On the Creation and Maintenance of Collective Memories: History as Social Psychology." In *Collective Memory of Political Events: Social Psychological Perspectives*, edited by James W. Pennebaker, Dario Paez, and Bernard Rimé, 3–19. Mahwah, NJ: Lawrence Erlbaum Associates, Publishers, 1997.

Proshansky, Harold M., Abbe K. Fabian, and Robert Kaminoff. "Place-Identity: Physical World Socialization of the Self." *Journal of Environmental Psychology* 3 (1983): 57–83.

Ricoeur, Paul. *Memory, History, Forgetting.* Translated by Kathleen Blamey and David Pellauer. Chicago: University of Chicago Press, 2004.

Rossi, Aldo. *The Architecture of the City.* Cambridge, MA: MIT Press, 2002.

Sato, Ikuya. *Fieldwork.* Tokyo: Shinyo-sha Publishing, 2006.

Shibazaki, T. *Yumemiru Shonen (A Dreaming Boy: Isamu Noguchi).* Sapporo: Kyoudoubunnkasha Publishing, 2005.

Stace, Walter T. *The Philosophy of Hegel.* New York: Dover, 1955.

Sturken, Marita. "The Aesthetics of Absence: Rebuilding Ground Zero." *American Ethnologist* 31, no. 3 (2004): 311–325.

Tanabe, M. *Boku No Ie Wa Koko Ni Atta (My House Was Here): A Record of Ground Zero Hiroshima.* Tokyo: Asahi-Shinbun Publishing, 2008.

Volkan, Vamik D. "Transgenerational Transmissions and "Chosen Trauma": An Element of Large-Group Identity." Paper presented at XIII International Congress International Association of Group Psychotherapy, 1998.

Werner, Heinz, and Bernard Kaplan. *Symbol Formation: An Organismic-Developmental Approach to Language and Thought.* New York: Psychology Press, 1984.

Whitehead, Alfred N. *Symbolism: Its Meaning and Effect (New Edition).* New York: Fordham University Press, 1985.

Yoneyama, Lisa. *Hiroshima Traces: Time, Space, and the Dialectics of Memory.* Berkeley: University of California Press, 1999.

Zolberg, Vera L. "Contested Remembrance: The Hiroshima Exhibit Controversy." *Theory and Society* 27, no. 4 (1998): 565–590.

# Memory Foundations

## Daniel Libeskind

**F**rom the beginning, I called my master plan for the World Trade Center site *Memory Foundations* because I felt that the key to the site was memory of September 11, 2001. At the same time, I felt that this event, this tragedy, should also be the foundation for twenty-first-century New York and for moving New York forward using memory as a bedrock of meaning for what happened on that tragic day. So memory and the future and memory and the affirmation of life were the key to transforming a disastrous site into a civic space, a space that really is for the people of New York.

### Developing the Master Plan

I did not start my project by thinking about buildings. I started with a singular fact: Nothing should be built where the tragedy took place. But that's easier said than done. When you have 10 million square feet of density plus many other programs that, together, have the density of a huge urban center (equivalent to the city of Baltimore or Denver) on a sixteen-acre site, the pressure is on to put many buildings on the site. But I considered it impossible to treat the World Trade Center site as a piece of real estate. This is the site where people perished.

*Designing the Site*

I decided very early that nothing should be built except the memorial and a civic space at the very center of the site, which is about half of the

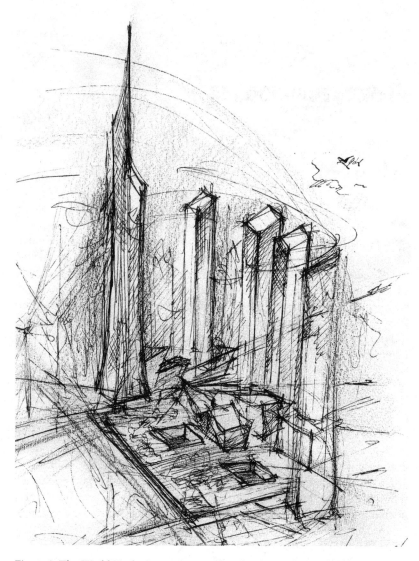

Figure 1. The World Trade Center Master Plan sketch. Credit: Daniel Libeskind

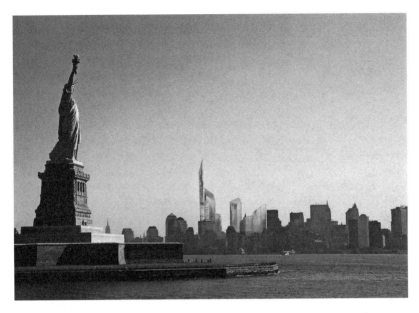

Figure 2. The World Trade Center in relation to the Statue of Liberty. Credit:
Daniel Libeskind

sixteen-acre site. And then how do you achieve the rest of the program-
ming? We have five towers, and even tower number two is taller than the
Empire State Building. We have an amazing number of massive buildings.
I put them on the periphery of the site. I wanted to bring a number of
symbolic aspects to the site so that the memorial would not only be a
shallow memorial at ground level, but that space would be available to the
public. I felt that only the experience of the totality of the site, including
the slurry wall, a huge retaining wall that was not designed to be seen,
would be part of the visitor experience.

I arranged the five buildings in a spiral formation to echo the torch of
the Statue of Liberty, which is just to the south. On the right hand side
of my competition drawing, you can see the footprints down below at
the bedrock level and the slurry wall rising to the left. This design goes
down seventy-five feet to bedrock. Early drawings include the slurry wall
and a building matrix.

These early sketches capture my early experiences of the site before
the competition was judged. There were many pragmatic considerations
for the site. Many people do not know, for example, that trains were run-

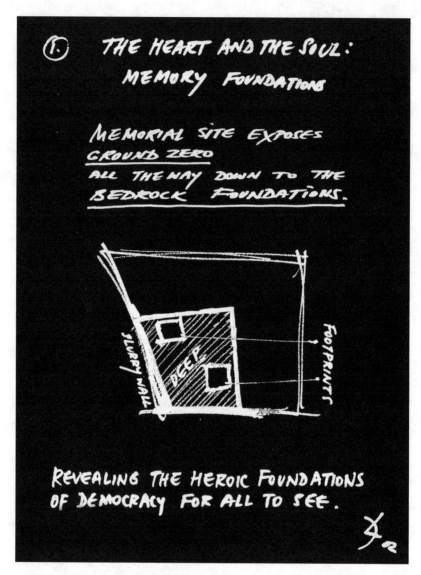

Figure 3. World Trade Center competition sketch 1, *The Heart and the Soul: Memory Foundations*. Credit: Daniel Libeskind

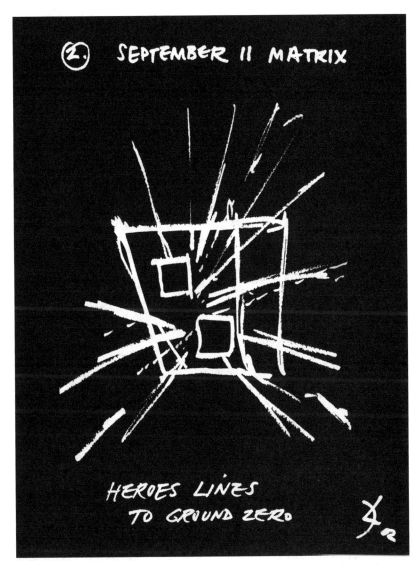

Figure 4. World Trade Center competition sketch 2, *September 11 Matrix*. Credit: Daniel Libeskind

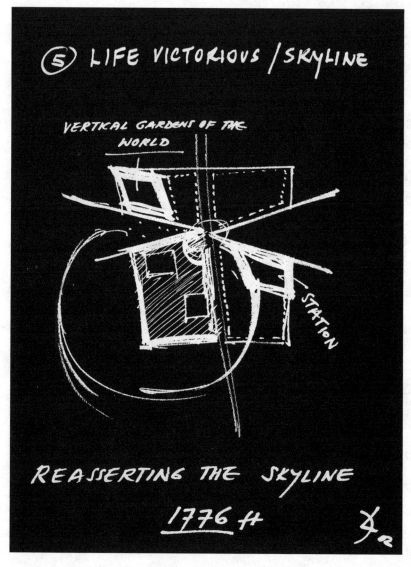

Figure 5. World Trade Center competition sketch 5, *Life Victorious/Skyline*. Credit: Daniel Libeskind

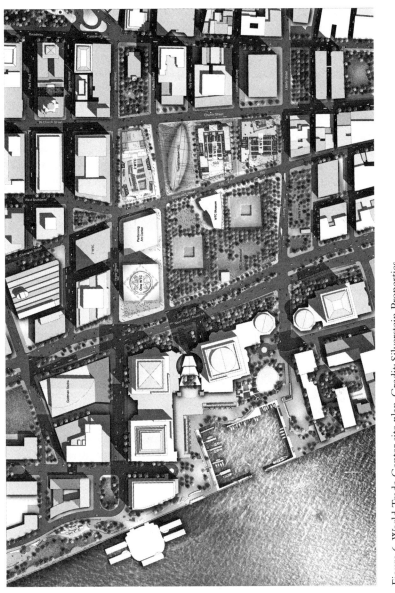

Figure 6. World Trade Center site plan. Credit: Silverstein Properties

ning underneath the World Trade Center site as the site was being constructed. The heart of New York City transportation—PATH trains and connections to subways—lie within this site. Thus, this is a special and dynamic site, and I wanted to make sure that civic space and memory are central to it.

In my site plan with all the key components, you see the footprints, the visitors' center, and the civic space. The slurry wall, which extends down to the bedrock, is part of the experience of visiting the footprints of the two towers. You see tower numbers one, two, three, four, and five surrounding the site in an emblematic formation. This is very large space, almost the size of San Marco in Venice. I felt that there would be many people coming from Broadway and the east side of Manhattan, so this is not a standalone site. It is a site that links Chinatown, Tribeca, Battery Park, and Wall Street. It has to work for the city as connective tissue.

## Wedge of Light

An extra triangle in the master plan is what I call the *Wedge of Light*. It is an additional public space determined by the two historic times: the light of that day at 8:46 a.m., when the tragedy began, and at 10:28 a.m., when the second tower collapsed. This is memory etched in light. The line of light at 10:28 moves us toward the memorial. Even on a non–9/11 day, the torsion of light created by the Wedge is haunting in some way. This experience is a component of a healing process, consistent with what the site strives to be. The Wedge of Light also serves as an entry point for the master plan. From an urbanistic perspective, this entry point brings an important historical site, St. Paul's Chapel, into the composition as you look outward toward Broadway. St. Paul's is the site where George Washington prayed for the nation's future in 1789, and after the trauma of the September 11 attacks, too, St Paul's was an important site. It was where people went to find others or experience solace. It is therefore a key point in the master plan.

## Slurry Wall

The Slurry Wall was not an element of the plan that was easy to achieve because exposing a living foundation is difficult. Engineers tell you that you have to put weight on top of it. But I felt that this emptiness, an emptiness in which so many lives were lost, conveys the visceral feeling of emptiness I had when I went down to the site. This was the key for me,

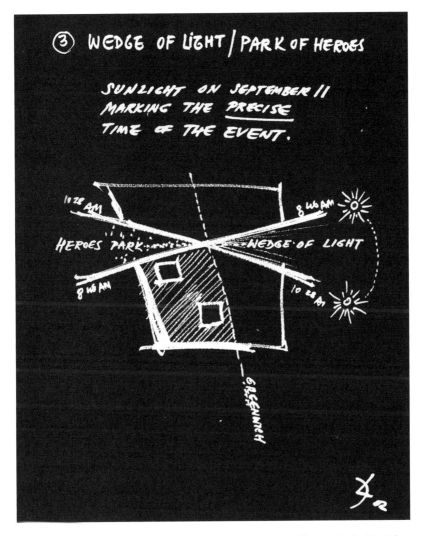

Figure 7 World Trade Center competition sketch 4, *Wedge of Light*. Credit: Daniel Libeskind

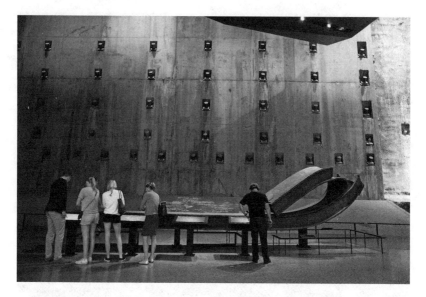

Figure 8. Slurry wall and signage steel at the World Trade Center Memorial Museum. Credit: Jin Lee

so I designed public access to it. The Slurry Wall is a moving and central part of the experience at the September 11 Memorial and Museum.

*Memorial Waterfalls*

The Memorial site is a very important element of the master plan. In my master plan I proposed a huge waterfall that would be vertical, the size of the footprints. There were many articles about this design in the news. A headline in the *New York Post,* "A Waterfall at the WTC?" ridiculed the idea of waterfalls in Lower Manhattan and described it as noisy and ridiculous: "How can you bring Niagara Falls to the memorial?"

But Michael Arad's design does exactly that. He brought his design for the two memorial pools to ground level, a beautiful idea that permitted connections between the World Trade Center site and the neighborhoods that were so badly affected by the September 11 attack. And he brought to life a key interest of mine: to include water as an important element. The intent of this was not only symbolic but also practical, since it would screen out the busy sounds of Lower Manhattan. It would offer solitude so that people in the future can talk and laugh and do anything, but it would still afford a sense of intimacy for those visiting the Memorial. Michael Arad's memorial works beautifully. When you stand and talk to somebody near at the names at the Memorial perimeter, you don't hear anything else because of the sound of those waterfalls. The sound, which is very forceful, creates a kind of an emptiness that was fundamental to the idea of the memorial.

*Buildings on the Site*

I fought for the 1,776-foot tower height of tower one. Port Authority of New York and New Jersey, the site's owner, asked: "How tall is the building?" But I wasn't interested in how many stories high the building was, and I couldn't care less about the tallest building in the world. That was not my interest. I wanted to create a building that has significance. When you look at the skyline from the bedrock of this tragedy, you are looking up, not just at an abstraction, but you're looking up at a date in the sky: 1776 is at this apex because the Declaration of Independence is, in many ways, a document that speaks about liberty and life itself. This, I thought, is the appropriate message for a high building that anchors the site's spiral.

I also fought for visitor platforms at the height of the former World Trade Center and for a small footprint for the buildings. Developers always want as large a footprint as possible to make the buildings more profitable. I was concerned that if tower one were a very large building, it would consume much of the public space. I therefore located it toward the Hudson River, where it would not throw shadows onto the memorial. Throughout the process, I thought about the quality of space and the appearance of the buildings as visitors looked toward the memorial, attuned to how the buildings act compositionally and how they speak.

*Preserving Public Space*

In my design for the master plan, I did everything possible to define the site and increase the amount of public space. Here's why: My parents were Holocaust survivors who became sweatshop workers in New York City. My father worked in a printing shop in a rat-infested building on Stone Street. If my parents were alive, they would never be in the towers. Nor would they have even entered the lobby of those towers, nor would they have entered shops on Church Street. Instead, they'd be on the streets of New York; they'd be in the subways; they'd be on the PATH trains. So I focused on what would people of New York City who would not be in the towers get from the redeveloped site. My strategy was to increase public space and to create a demand for civic architecture. The master plan did not treat streets and the PATH station as mere parts of the transportation system but as integral elements of the plan. The site of the World Trade Center is not a business-as-usual site, though it must also work as business as usual.

*Planning as a Democratic Process*

A rendering of the site gives one true faith in the democratic process. Democracy is very difficult. A lot of people told me, "Mr. Libeskind, you should get out of this process. Nothing is going to happen. You're compromising. Forget about it." Democracy can take hard work. Trying to link up diverse interests can also be hard work. The interests of the developers are totally different from the interests of families and people on the street. Yet, though these interests are all very different, bringing them together is important.

The site, with all its elements, has passed through many different hands. When you design a master plan, you're providing an image and a structure for it to be filled in by many talented people. Michael Arad's memorial is fantastic, and the museum is now complete.

## The Master Plan's Influence in Lower Manhattan

While I was designing the master plan, it was quite controversial. There were many voices and many critiques: "The memorial is too big," "The buildings are too close to each other," or "What about the _____?" There were many competing interests and compromises along the way as we were working with many stakeholders: families of the victims; the Port Authority of New York and New Jersey, the site's owner, a gigantic organization run by governors of New York and New Jersey; the governor of New York State; the mayor of New York City; PATH authorities that control PATH trains between New York City and New Jersey; the Metropolitan Transit Authority, New York City's subway system; as well as every person in New York City. Everyone was saying, "This is a compromise!" The project, therefore, was not just about an idea; it was also about creating a consensus, a plan that could move forward. Yet I am amazed that despite these disparate voices, how close the realization of the Ground Zero Master Plan came to my original drawings.

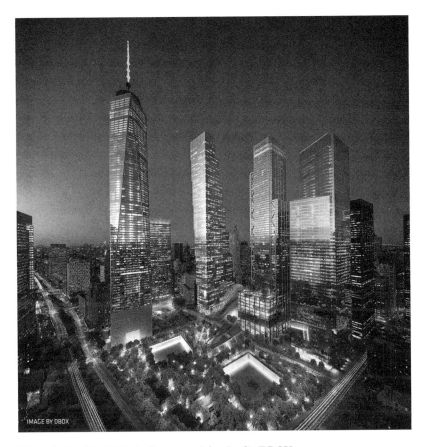

Figure 9. The World Trade Center at night. Credit: DBOX

## Streets

As an example of details that have influence but are unnoticed, I spent much of my time with technicians and the Port Authority discussing, for example, whether we can make a street two inches wider. This is a design issue that was not in the newspapers. It is not a glamorous task, but it is a fundamental thing that we take for granted. We walk, and the street is just two inches wider. It is very difficult to get those two inches, maybe more difficult than making a large building, because you're tampering with so many agencies that control this space and have their own requirements and ideas. A sidewalk is that kind of almost-invisible aspect of the city that we may feel but not realize.

I learned about the fundamental importance of sidewalks in Berlin when I was living there during the construction of the Jewish Museum. The names of all the streets changed many times. They changed during Hitler's time, then they changed again when the Soviets occupied Berlin, then they changed again after the unification of East and West Berlin. But something that didn't change was the sidewalks. The street names changed, but the sidewalks remained as they always were. Even when the city was bombed during World War II, the one thing you still saw was the outline of the streets.

Streets are important as they are about public space. They are about the way people walk, the way they congregate, and the way they connect socially. I often thought about this because in this era of information technology, social space is especially important. We have many illusions about what it means to be social—such as giving our opinion on a blog, but the Internet is not in fact a social medium. A social medium allows us to be with other people on the street, to talk to somebody, to look at somebody, to have an accidental conversation or overhear something and get engaged. That is the power of the Ground Zero site—the streets and spaces that bring people together.

*Change in Lower Manhattan*

I am amazed at the fundamental changes this plan brought to Lower Manhattan, changes we could not have expected in 2011. Hundreds of thousands of people have moved to Lower Manhattan and use the public space that was created. The site has regenerated an ancient area of New York City in a way that no one expected. When I was working on this project at its inception, I said that by the time these buildings are built, Wall Street will not work the same as it does today. And so it happened. Most occupants of the new towers are not connected with Wall Street but, instead, there are many creative media companies occupying the towers. The articulation of the master plan—with its spatial relationships among light and things that we do not even see because they are below ground—by a fantastic group of architects that worked on this project has made this site a new epicenter of New York City. It has changed the way people think about this area, which was so often a gloomy area at night. Now retail is moving in along with hotels and all sorts of things.

*The Master Plan in Retrospect*

I think very few people could understand how complex this project is. After all, it's not a building, it's not a memorial, it's not a museum, it's not a piazza, it's not a green space. It's a piece of the city. To me, that is the project's core: to build a piece of the city. That is a much more difficult project than building a building. It is much more difficult than building a park. It is much more difficult than building a monument. We had to come together at the right time to do the right things—and we did.

A master plan is a very precise instrument, not a vague fantasy. You have to draw all the lines and all the relationships. It is like a musical score. At first, a musical score is very abstract without an orchestra or musicians. It just looks like some dots on lines because it needs to be performed. The performance is not just the violin and cello, it is also the back of the conductor. I always say my back is to the audience because I'm not this tower or that tower. It is also like a musical score because you have to be able to give very precise instructions, but you also have to give freedom of interpretation. Without that, it is a mechanical performance and a failure. It is that balance between designing the master plan and the interpretations of the master plan that is now realized. And it is not yet over. There will be new things happening around the site: new buildings, streets, and shops. It is a magnet of development, but also a magnet for the rethinking of social space, urban space, economic space, and aesthetic space. As it develops further, it will change New York in many ways that we cannot now foresee.

*Ancient Remnants and the Natural Environment at the Site*

When construction began on the World Trade Center site, workers found a wooden boat from the seventeenth century. This is the beauty of cities: They have a history, a truth, and that truth is not somebody's invention. Instead, it is embodied in city space in traces of the city's evolution that remains from the past and continues into the future.

My plan took the history of that site very seriously, going back to before New York was New York. The water is particularly important because of the fact that the city is on an island. It's not a coincidence that I originally thought of waterfalls. It seemed to me that water is a key, and not just for the acoustic sense of dampening the traffic sound, but also as water. Water gave birth to Manhattan as ships came in and the island was discovered by both Native peoples and later by generations of Europeans. You cannot separate the symbolic from the practical in a city because everything is entwined, and everything has a meaning because people live here. In New York City, nature has become part of our culture.

Therefore, this site needed to be created from the ground up through its traces. This is also how this city developed. We still have a Broad Street, a Stone Street, a Liberty Street, and a Church Street. Even their names offer orientation. I always thought about a circle of light, which is central to the site's design. Even though the buildings are standing in a grid, they are responding to a torchlike movement around the site because they are on the very periphery of Ground Zero. I pushed the buildings as far away from the public space to have as much light as possible there; that was my idea of the torch of liberty. Even in today's political climate when people are renouncing symbols of freedom and liberty, the symbols are there at the site to be experienced.

What is important is that people can feel these symbols in a breath of air, in the view across to the Hudson River. They can feel a balance of the scheme, where the towers are standing, and how they're framing the site. I tried to imbue the site with those things. This is why people like the site. They understand that it is for them, that it is their site. They can interpret it as they wish as they walk through it.

On my daily visits to the site, I sometimes stand next to a name I don't know and talk with somebody. Sometimes they have been visitors; sometimes somebody is related to the person named; sometimes somebody accidentally stumbled upon the site—and that's what makes that site unique. You can sit on a bench or go to the shopping center; you can go underground; you can be in the terminal; you can be in the World Financial Center. Each of these venues has meaning. The World Trade Center site is part of city so it has regular city functions, but there is also something celebratory about it, even though it is a place where something terrible happened.

*What Is a Master Plan?*

There is no project more complex than a master plan. There can't be, because there's no instruction book for this. Maybe in retrospect one can learn lessons from it; can study it; can see the politics, the economics, and the aesthetics. The process of this project was completely different than the design of the original World Trade Center in 1978–79, which was a top-down process. The Port Authority of New York and New Jersey decided on the project, Minoru Yamasaki designed it, and when people woke up they saw those two towers. They loved or hated them, but it didn't matter, because the project was done. But this is a different era. This project ushered in an era of public participation. One of the biggest aspects of the design competition and the interest and controversies it generated was the awareness that people are the core of the city, and people should make decisions. They should participate in their own city's design.

*The Public Spirit*

Ultimately, the spirit of the site is the public spirit. It was designed to give the public access, not as a singular gesture, but to make it a work in-the-round from the Hudson River, from the East River, from Battery Park, from Wall Street, from Tribeca, from Chinatown. For all the neighborhoods that were here right along, this became a center. And it continues to change. It takes a while because there is no housing developed as part of the project—it is office buildings, cultural facilities, and site infrastructure—but people are coming because they want to be here and be part of this. Within this rebirth set in motion by the site, there is a feeling of dynamism. I see many schools and families that have little to do with Wall Street here. This is a neighborhood that has taken off. I'm amazed, because when I first started this project some people were very pessimistic and thought this area would never come back—and yet it has.

I think this project also changed the world. Whether you are in London, Singapore, or Europe there is no longer the possibility of doing a large-scale, high-density project without consulting the public. The public will challenge the project: "What is happening? Who decided this? Who hired these developers? Who decided how tall these buildings would be?" I think this project was the beginning of this change. We are seeing it incrementally, but I think that in retrospect we will see it as a change in the way people see their cities and their role in shaping it.

## Autobiographical Reflections

I was an immigrant to New York from Poland via Israel. Like millions of others who came to America before planes were cheaper than boats, I stood on deck of the ship at 5:00 a.m. with my sister and stared at the city. I had an incredible and indelible feeling of coming to America, to New York. And that feeling was in my heart as I descended into the bedrock of the World Trade Center site: I saw that boat; I saw all those immigrants; I saw my grandmother; I saw myself, my mother, my sister; and I saw the Statue of Liberty and what it represents. I saw the skyline

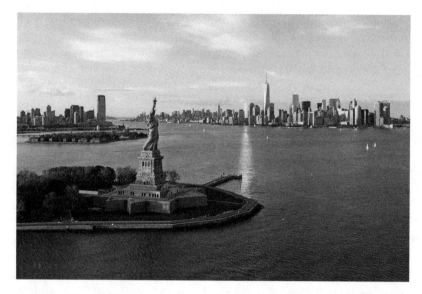

Figure 10. The World Trade Center as seen from a helicopter. Credit: Joe Woolhead

of New York, which is the most unbelievable skyline as you see it from the water because it is the proof of liberty, of diversity, of individuality, of ambition—of everything that America and New York stand for in terms of freedom and power for the poor, for the immigrants, for the lower classes. That was what this project was about for me.

The press and people often ask me where I was on September 11. I was living in Berlin at that time with my family in order to build the Jewish Museum. It took thirteen years for that museum to be built for many reasons, including politics. On the morning of September 11 I went to my studio and turned to my friends, my wife, and my partners and said, "You know, this is a great day for me. The museum project is complete. I don't have to think about Jewish history or German history. I can now go to the office and do something else because now people can enter the museum and they can see for themselves." And then, around 2:30 p.m. Berlin time, we saw those images on the screens. I suddenly realized that you can never say that some part of history is finished. Histories are strangely interlinked.

Memory and the future are also interlinked, and that was what the master plan was about. It was about how to bring the affirmation of life to life—the affirmation of what we stand for as New Yorkers, as Americans, and as free people around the world. It was about how to take that memory of this tragic event that murdered Americans as well as people from many, many countries. It was about how to use that space in a way that is sensitive, that is significantly civic, but that is also a space that works for the future of New York. How will it be a space for new generations who have only read about these attacks as well as for those for whom 9/11 was a visceral, tragic experience? The memorial and museum are so moving because they are a visceral experience, not just an intellectual one. Nor do they evoke only the images we saw immediately after 9/11. It is the feeling that your soul, your heart, your whole personality, and your individuality is implicated in a memory and in a resoluteness of what it means for the good of New York, for the good of the world, and for the good of freedom.

# Building the 9/11 Memorial

## Michael Arad

The process of thinking about the design of the September 11 Memorial started a few months after the attacks. I was here in New York on the day of the attacks and was incredibly affected by what I had seen and, more important, what followed that day—the way that New Yorkers came together in the wake of that attack with remarkable courage and compassion. The attacks brought people together and showed us the best of humankind in the wake of the worst. That is what compelled me to start thinking about a design for a memorial.

## Initial Design Ideas

I originally thought about a memorial that would be out in the Hudson River. I thought of the surface of the river being torn open, forming two voids, with water flowing into these voids. It was an enigmatic image—something that doesn't make sense, since water doesn't behave that way. But that image persisted and haunted me. I ended up building a small model over the course of the next year that captured that sense—the surface of the water being torn open and forming two square voids in the river water with the river rushing in and onto itself. Ultimately, the two voids would come to represent the sense of persistent absence. Eventually I took that little model and photographed it on the rooftop of my apartment building. And then I set it aside. I could see the absence of the towers in the skyline of Manhattan that reflected in the surface of the water in these two empty voids (Figure 1).

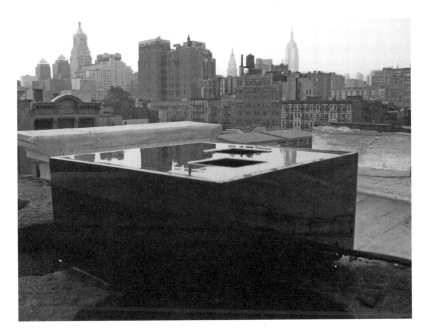

Figure 1. Initial model. Credit: Michael Arad

I spent a year on this process, a year that was a cathartic and very private investigation. I came back to it after the selection of the master plan for the redevelopment of the World Trade Center site. I felt that Daniel Libeskind's master plan, unlike most other plans, reintegrated the site back into the life of the city. It brought Greenwich and Fulton Streets through the site and subdivided the sixteen-acre site into four unequal quadrants. The largest quadrant, measuring close to eight acres, would be where the towers once stood.

I wanted to take that cue created by the master plan—this notion of tying the site back into the life of the city—and go even further with it. The master plan suggested a site some thirty feet below street level. I thought: Let's bring it up to grade. Let's link it to the surrounding streets and sidewalks of the city in ways that are similar to what you see at Union Square or Washington Square. I drew on those precedents and other plazas located elsewhere in the city based on my firsthand knowledge of experiencing those sites in the weeks that followed the attack.

If you think of Union Square, you might think of the farmers' market. If you think of Washington Square, you might think of kids strumming a guitar near its central fountain. But in the days that followed the attack, these places, street corners, the public realm, were especially important. These were spaces that allowed us to come together and to support one another in meaningful ways. These places didn't just bring us together physically; they also brought us together as a community. They allowed us to offer help and compassion to others and, in turn, to receive that same gesture.

I also developed an idea after visiting a quarry in South Orange, New Jersey. Something about the precise geometry of the material being removed and its sense of ruin and renewal appealed to me greatly. Water, vegetation, and rubble were all mixed together. These ideas launched me and led to sketches that tried to bring the idea of the voids in the Hudson River to the site. This led to my creating the two large voids in a flat, urban plaza for my competition entry (Figure 2).

The last few words that describe my design for the memorial said "residents on their way to work or play." I understood "play" as an important and unlikely word to end on. This site had to become a living part of New York City as well as a profound site for memory. This suggested bringing the plaza up to grade, carving out the two voids, and creating memorial galleries to surround the voids where visitors would encounter the names of victims. I understood that the moment of coming up to the site would be a powerful and difficult moment. It would be a moment of comprehension, from seeing the scale of the tower's footprints being echoed in the memorial, seeing the size of the void in the middle of the city, and seeing the multitude of names that would surround each footprint.

## Developing the Memorial's Design

When I came to the site designated for the memorial in 2003 as one of eight finalists, I saw the slurry wall and thought we could find a way to preserve that wall and exhibit it—perhaps not in open air but within a memorial museum—where the memorial plaza could serve as its roof. At the lowest basement slab seventy feet below the surrounding street level, I saw the cut-off columns that had been exposed by recovery efforts. They remained from the steel columns that had connected each tower to its foundation. Seeing these traces of the towers, the slurry wall, and the torch-cut columns on that first visit, I was struck by the power of these artifacts. I realized that we do not need to reconstruct these towers because we can imagine them by the traces they left behind. The memorial design was not about re-creating what had been, but about making that absence present, and visible, and tangible.

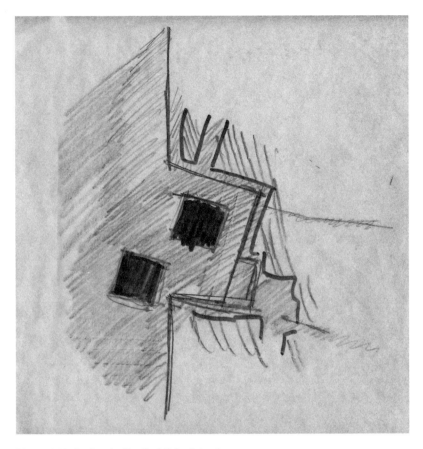

Figure 2. Early sketch. Credit: Michael Arad

The visit to site informed my final competition entry, in which I described the memorial plaza I proposed as both a prologue to and epilogue of the experience of coming up to the edge of the voids. I also described the importance of linking this site to the life of the city by bringing the site up to grade in order to link it to the streets and sidewalks nearby.

*Abacus Bands of Trees*

When I showed my images and model to the jury, its members expressed concern that though the model physically linked the memorial to the

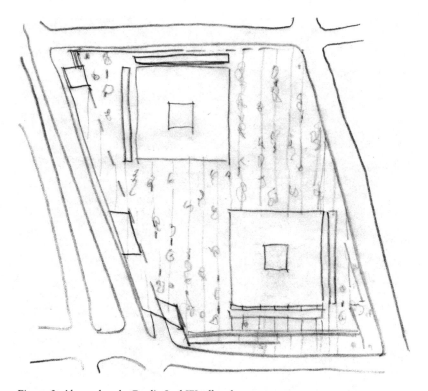

Figure 3. Abacus bands. Credit: Joel Woolhead

city, it still felt austere, as if the site was dedicated solely to memorial uses. They pushed me to integrate the site into the life of the city, as I had described in my presentation. They thought that the landscape elements on the site—seventy or eighty tall eastern white pine trees placed on the site—did not do enough to bring that sense of life back to the site. This challenged me to think about how could I take this landscape design and alter it in order to address that concern. I was concerned that a very strong pattern or a very bold figure in the landscape design would compete with the clarity of that first design gesture of the flat plane of the two voids.

I struggled with this question for a few weeks and I came up with an idea I called *abacus-like bands*, a series of paving bands that could unify this memorial plaza and its material treatment (Figure 3). Some of these bands would be wide; others would be narrow. Along the length of the bands, almost like beads traveling along the wires of an abacus, trees could be placed at random intervals. So there would be a soft underlying order to the design. If you looked east or west you would see the trees snap into these long rows. But if you looked north or south, the clarity of that geometry would dissipate and you would see a staggered, naturalistic placement of trees.

The jury approved my design in early 2004, and we went to work on realizing it and all of its details. These details including questions we had not been considering before: Where were the bathrooms and the information desk? Where would school groups queue? How would we actually build the waterfall? What kind of waterfall would it be? Would it be like Paley Park, where you have the water falling on the surface of a wall? A wall that would be canted slightly to allow that to happen would require much more water and a rusticated surface. Or would we do something similar to the fountain at the World Financial Center where the water could freefall over the edge of the weir? That is what we ended up doing.

*Waterfalls*

We constructed a mockup of the corner of one of the pools in Canada in our fountain designer's backyard and tested various profiles for weir serrations from winter through the summer of 2005 (Figure 4). We often complain about the design process: how long it is and how difficult it is. But it is an absolutely necessary process because the process enriches the design. It is through the development of these details that the clarity of an idea comes to the foreground.

The design of the weir gave us the opportunity to bring the idea of both individual loss and collective loss into an element of the design that had not been considered before. The clarity of individual strands of water dissipates as the water falls thirty feet down. By the time the water is halfway down the waterfall, it is no longer possible to see individual strands. Instead, there is a tapestry-like curtain of falling water. This idea was not there in the onset, but it was driven by the clear idea of acknowledging both individual and collective loss, an idea that was there from the start.

*Memorial Galleries*

The memorial galleries were an important part of the design. They were intended to shelter that moment of encountering the names, a very difficult and vulnerable moment of taking in the magnitude and scale of what had happened at this site. I had been struck by an iconic photograph in *Daily News* on the 2006 anniversary of 9/11, in which a uniformed firefighter knelt at the edge of one of these temporary pools. Something about that image captured me. I imagined that type of reverence occurring here.

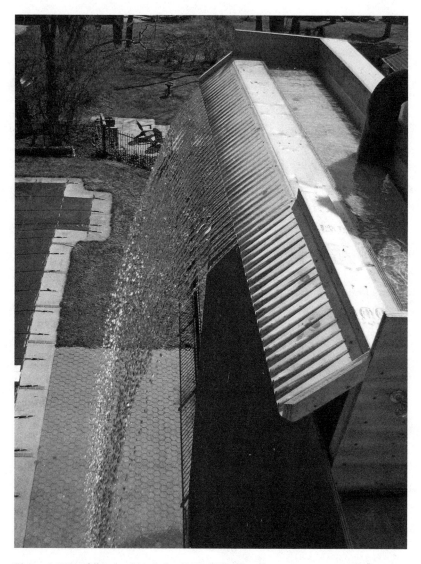

Figure 4. Waterfall in backyard. Credit: Joel Woolhead

In the years after the attacks, temporary memorial pools were built every year at Ground Zero for family members to gather around as they descended to the site. So that was what I expected people to do at these memorial galleries I had envisioned, a cloister-like space surrounding each void. There would be a moment of communion with the names that I felt had to be sheltered. But for a variety of reasons having to do with budget, security, and apprehensions family members felt about descending some thirty feet below the plaza to stand at the edge of the voids, we were asked to bring the names up to plaza level. Initially, I felt apprehensive about that change.

Over the next few years we went through a long process of trying to find the right way of re-creating that moment at the edge of the void, a threshold and a dividing line. One idea was to end the plaza, begin a water table, and have the letters break the surface of the water like thousands of small islands. The water would cascade into the void beyond them. Another idea was to create a bronze sculptural shape that would ring the voids. Water would well up at the very top of that vessel. After testing dozens and dozens of ideas, we were able to recapture that moment, not within memorial galleries but up at street level and firmly within the city.

What you see now at the memorial is an eight-foot-wide water table that is two feet high. It rings the voids and serves as the spring point for the waterfalls. Above that are bronze panels suspended over this water table with a five-sided profile, almost like a wing, that has been incised with names of the victims. These names appear as shadows during the day as a result of the materials that have been removed from that half-inch-thick bronze plate. At night, the wing is illuminated from within, and the names appear as lights.

*Placement of Names*

The placement of the names was one of the most challenging issues to resolve. How would we arrange the names of the victims around the memorial? It was not a question I dealt with until after the design was selected. It was a question I grappled with for a long time. One idea was to recognize first responders with an insignia next to their name. A Maltese cross, the symbol of the New York Fire Department, could perhaps be placed next to the name of a fire fighter. That idea was rejected at the time as too honorific by some and not sufficient by others.

I then suggest an approach I called *meaningful adjacency*. There would be a reason why one name is next to another. I did not want to create alphabetical listing. Something that felt like a ledger seemed inappropriate. We wanted to give primacy to a sense of individual loss, and what a better way to capture that than through a person's name? Not a person's name and the floor they worked on and the company they worked for or their age, but that person's name. I proposed that we reach out to the close to three thousand families involved and ask if there are names of other victims that they would like to see placed next to the name of the person that they lost. Doing so would allow these personal connections to come into the design of the memorial. Family members could be next to one another whether or not they shared the same last name, whether they were married or not. Friends, coworkers, and people who had gone to school together or had commuted together every day could be next to one another.

When I first suggested this idea, it was seen as onerous to implement and logistically difficult. It was therefore rejected and set aside. I couldn't come up with another idea other than literally letting chance dictate the placement of every name so that it would be equitable. Even something as simple as an alphabetical listing carries weight to it. Two men with the name, Michael Francis Lynch, perished that day. The idea of having those two names side by side—without any way of distinguishing which name belonged to which person because they were the same name—just felt wrong. We also had family members that shared the same last name but others that didn't. So I suggested a brutal but fair idea of a haphazard listing of the names. That upset many family members, and I understand why. In response, they came together with another way of arranging the names. It was suggested that people be listed along with the company they worked for, the tower they perished in, the floor number, and their age. That created what looked like a directory. I didn't want the names stacked in columns; I wanted each name to be staggered individually to give each of them a unique geographic space that emphasized that sense of individuality rather than being part of a list.

In 2006, when Mayor Michael Bloomberg became chair of the Memorial Foundation, this was one of the first questions he wanted to address. We discussed this at length at Gracie Mansion. As is well known, Bloomberg is a very data-driven guy, and he came to this conversation with a lot of information already in his grasp. We decided to modify the arrangement into nine broad categories reflecting where people were that day: on the four flights, in the two towers, at the Pentagon, the 1993 bombing victims, and the first responders. And the first responders, in turn, were also grouped by where they came from that day: the same firehouse, the same precinct building. But within these groups—and some of these groups have over a thousand names in them—the names could be arranged according to meaningful adjacency. The mayor accepted that idea, which was remarkably brave for somebody in political office because there was no sense of how successful we would be in actually implementing that idea. As could easily be imagined, we might be able to meet half of the requests but not the other half.

We got more than 1,200 requests and spent over a year arranging the names very carefully to implement this idea. We were eventually able to meet all the requests, which felt like a great achievement. It allowed us to bring meaning into the design that we wouldn't be able to do independently; it had to be a process that solicited this information. Now you have siblings side by side—but you also have other people who are side by side (Figure 5).

You wouldn't know what connects two people if you hadn't gone through this process. For example, one young woman lost her father that day on Flight 11. She also lost her best friend from college who was working in the North Tower when Flight 11 crashed into it. Her father's name is among the last under "Flight 11," her friend's name is close to it, among the first under "Word Trade Center." The number—close to three thousand dead—is very hard to relate to. By breaking it down into individual stories, we can build a partial understanding of what happened that day to so many families. By doing that, every time you come back to the memorial you might focus on a different story. You might have a greater appreciation for the impact that day had.

## Inauguration of the Memorial, 2011

The Memorial opened in September 2011. The site looks like a simple green square in the middle of the city (Figure 6), but it is anything but that.

Below the plaza are hundreds of thousands of square feet of program space. We have a museum, a train station, and a subway line. We have a pedestrian concourse, retail space, pump rooms, and a chiller plant. But all of that disappears from view. The experience is ultimately about being in a public space with a memorial plaza and two pools (Figure 7). At the center of each pool are voids and they are very much about connecting to the site's past. This is all within an eight-acre plaza that is very much part of New York.[1]

While working on the memorial, I wanted to imagine office workers coming here from across the street during their lunch breaks, neighborhood residents coming through here with their kids, and all these groups sharing this space (Figure 8). These public spaces reflect our values as a society and they can allow multiple activities to go on side by side. It is about looking to the past and marking absence.

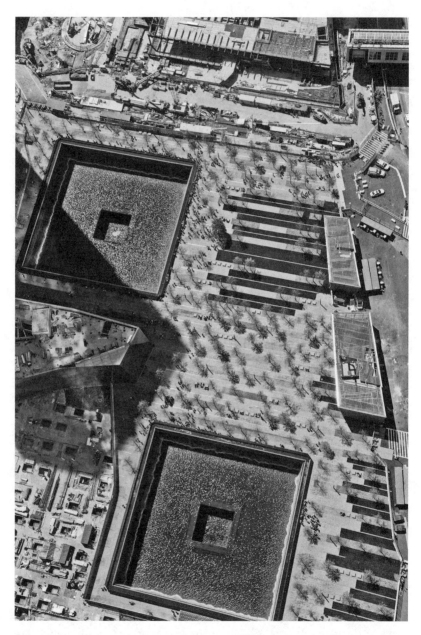

Figure 5. Work in progress, eight-acre site. Credit: Joe Woolhead

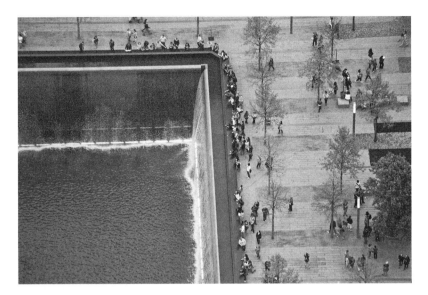

Figure 6. Pool with visitors. Credit: Joe Woolhead

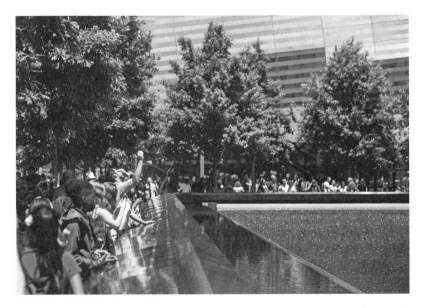

Figure 7. Shared space at south Memorial pool. Credit: Jin Lee, courtesy of National September 11 Memorial and Museum

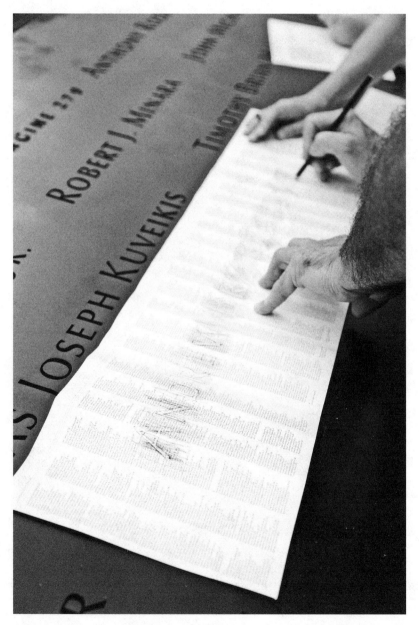

Figure 8. Names panel. Credit: Joe Woolhead

Everything we have done over the years—creating these waterfalls and name panels, planting these trees, and paving this plaza—was all about inanimate objects. The site came to life with people on September 11, 2011, in a remarkable way that was gratifying to see (Figure 8). As site construction has continued to be completed, more streets have opened, more trees were planted, and the site now welcomes people to a living part of New York City. To see kids running around the site while others are engaged in thought just a few feet away is a true affirmation of this vision.

## Changes at the Memorial Site

The most significant change since the memorial opened in September 2011 has been how the urban context around the site has started to fill in (Figure 9).

We opened the memorial before the surrounding streets and sidewalks were completed. Visiting the memorial then entailed a ticket process and going through security screening. Connecting the memorial site to the city was a driving force in my design: to make the memorial part of the urban fabric of New York City. With fences all around and ticketing and security screening in 2011, that was not coming through.

### Opening the Site

Opening the site to the public was a gradual process. It began at the southeast corner of the memorial at the corner of Liberty and Church. The fence came down there without any announcement. With jersey barriers and fences removed, all of a sudden all of New York started walking in. Our office is not far away, so I ran down and took photos of people walking to the memorial without the rigmarole of ticketing and screening. It was very gratifying to see. In the years since, removal of fences and barriers has extended all the way around the memorial plaza. This has not only changed the memorial but has also changed who is there in a significant way. It is no longer just people who are there to visit the memorial. Now we have people who work and live there using the site as well. If you go to the site early in the morning, you see commuters walking purposefully across the memorial. You see residents of the neighborhood on their way to school or to work, and at lunchtime you see a different group of people walking through (Figures 10, 11, and 12). That was always my vision for the memorial.

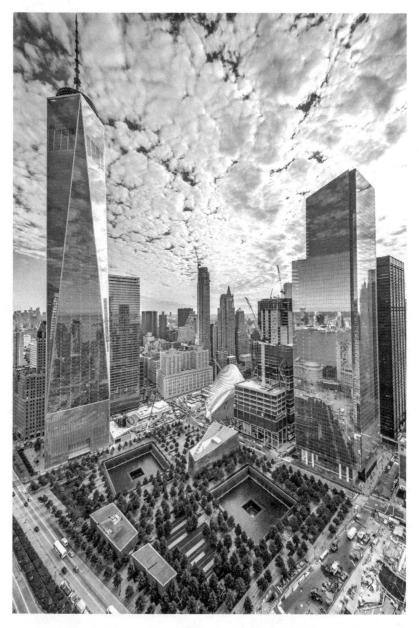

Figure 9. Memorial plaza and the World Trade Center site within Lower Manhattan.

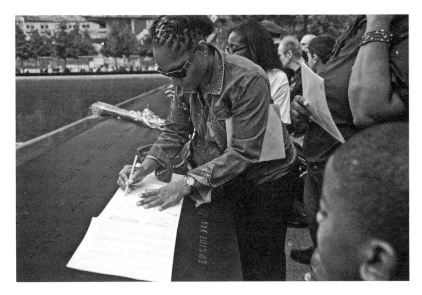

Figure 10. Woman at names panel. Credit: Joe Woolhead

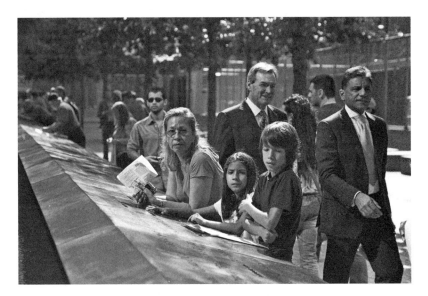

Figure 11. Names panel and businessmen. Credit: Joe Woolhead

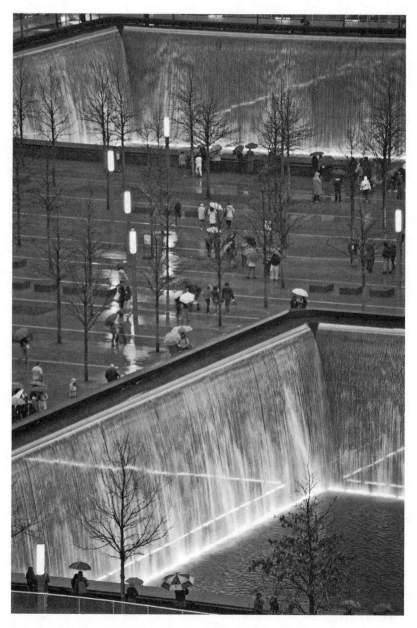

Figure 12. Night rain at the Memorial. Credit: Joe Woolhead

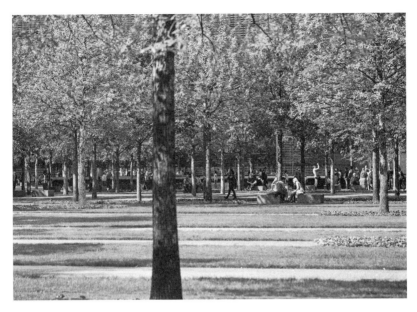

Figure 13. Mature tree canopy. Credit: Jin Lee, courtesy of National September 11 Memorial and Museum

*Trees*

Plantings on the plaza have also changed since 2011. Trees are maturing. The more mature trees are at the south end because of the sequence in which they were planted. Construction remained ongoing at the north end, but as this work is completed, fences come down and more trees are planted. Every year the memorial seems to be coming more into its own. Near the memorial visitors can now walk under a canopy of trees, this is now one of the largest open spaces in Lower Manhattan (Figure 13).

## Competing Interests

In a project of this scope, there are always competing interests. One example of this was when the PATH train station designers wanted to put skylights over the platform leading down to the train tracks. That area is directly below the memorial so there would be people standing above those skylights and the skylights would have been part of the memorial plaza. We would not have been able to plant any trees there, we would not have had paving there and that area would not have felt like it was part of the rest of the memorial plaza. If the PATH design were the only interest that was going to be represented, then there would have been skylights. It would have made for a great experience for people standing below those skylights, but that was not the only interest to consider. This exemplifies, for the whole project, how the process needed to include multiple voices. If one party controls much of what gets built on any single block, only their interests and point of view are going to get represented and built. Then everyone else has to live with that.

## Recognizing Victims of Toxic Exposure on the Plaza

One issue that has emerged in the years since the memorial opened is that it does not recognize rescuers, recovery workers, and others who became ill because of exposure to the toxins at the site. Hundreds have died, and, unfortunately, more will die because of the toxins at the site. Unlike the very definitive tally of 2,983 victims of the September 11 attack provided by the New York City Office of Chief Medical Examiner, there is no definitive tally—nor will there ever be—of all the people who suffered because of exposure to toxins: people who worked at the site, kids in local schools in the area, and residents who live there.

When I was finally brought into the room to hear these conversations, the thing that struck me the most was the sense that people who are a part of this community do not feel that there is a place on the memorial plaza that belongs to them. The memorial is dedicated to the people who died on September 11 and their families, so this community feels almost like interlopers on that plaza. It is terrible to hear that a space designed to be welcoming, supportive, and reflective feels as if it excludes the story of people who were profoundly affected by this attack.

We've been asked to look at adding an element to the design of the memorial that acknowledges the loss of life that is a longitudinal effect of the terrorist attack on September 11. It is a challenge because we have completed the design and the memorial is built. As this chapter is being written, we are trying to integrate something into the design that will address this pressing need. We are looking at changing the design at the southwest quadrant of the memorial starting at the corner of West and Liberty Streets and creating a path that runs diagonally north and east. It will utilize a clearing we had created that is underutilized because lawn beds that are interspersed with bands of stone paving could not be left open to the public on a regular basis. This is an opportunity to improve the design by creating a path that is roughly where the Ground Zero site access ramp stood that was used during the rescue and recovery effort. We are envisioning a series of stone monoliths—the same gray-green granite as the plaza—erupting out of the flat paving of the plaza. The monoliths, which might have markers with language (all of which is still under discussion), will define a path commemorating those who, as a consequence of the attack, later became ill or died.

I feel privileged to be doing this. This was an omission—not an intentional omission but an omission nonetheless—and we have an opportunity to right that wrong in a way that feels appropriate to the design of the rest of the memorial. The new path is not about a linear experience; it is about creating a place on the memorial plaza that is dedicated to people who became ill and died as a result of the attacks, a place where people can gather, a place that belongs to them. I hope it will feel that way.

## Concluding Thoughts

The memorial design changed in many ways over the eight years that I was involved in it. We had galleries underground, and then we didn't. The names moved from one place to another. But the two principles that propelled the memorial design forward did not change: creating an open, public, democratic space for gathering; and trying to make absence visible and tangible. Those were the core ideas at the heart of the design and they remained. They were articulated in different ways as things changed, but those ideas did not change.

The memorial represents a quiet defiance too, that a deadly and destructive terrorist attack cannot take away our life in the city and what it means to live in the city. There was a terrorist attack in October 2017 on the bike path close to the memorial that killed eight people. I made a point of biking to work the day that the bike path reopened. It was important for me to say, "This is our space." I've been on that bike path multiple times before, and I'm not going to stop using that bike path. I'm not going to change my life. The bike path is a small thing, but it is the larger principle: not letting the actions that were inflicted upon us change how we will be

### Note

1. A description of *Reflecting Absence* by architect Michael Arad and landscape architect Peter Walker can be found on the Lower Manhattan Development Corporation website at http://www.wtcsitememorial.org/fin7.html.

# Urban Security in New York City After 9/11
## Risk and Realities

Charles R. Jennings

he attacks of 9/11 were a turning point in governmental approaches
to securing urban areas. The declaration of a "Global War on Terror" and the concomitant mobilization of finances and resources by the
government have redefined the traditional divisions between private and
public security, and realigned the relationship between federal security
apparatuses and local governments in large urban areas. Of more local im-
port, the repercussions of 9/11 affected the historic relationship between
New York's largest public safety agencies—the New York Police Department (NYPD) and Fire Department of New York (FDNY). Over three
mayoral administrations, the effects of both these changes have impacted
everyday service delivery and assumed an important if unacknowledged
role in local politics and public administration.

In addition, the targeting of US-based civil targets by Al Qaeda linked
global relations and foreign policy to local risk more closely than ever
before. Decisions made by the federal government in the Global War on
Terror half a world away now have immediate impacts on business and
public security in the city. The "scale up" of federal domestic security,
notably through the formation of the Department of Homeland Security,
released unprecedented sums of direct state and local aid to ostensibly
improve public safety and resistance to terrorist attacks. New York City is
both the exemplar and the outlier in the adoption of a "homeland security" orientation among America's local law enforcement agencies.

In the weeks and months that followed, New York City, led in large
measure by the NYPD, began to reinvent itself with an orientation toward

counterterrorism. The NYPD, as of 2001, had achieved large reductions in crime, and was well regarded for its methods and techniques. Over the following ten-plus years, coinciding with the election of Michael Bloomberg, who succeeded Rudolph Giuliani as mayor, the NYPD underwent remarkable change. The confluence of the emphasis on crime reduction, the new focus on preventing terrorist attacks, and a remarkably permissive oversight climate by elected officials and the media jointly enabled an unprecedented series of developments in the city's law enforcement that would place the NYPD in a unique position among local law enforcement agencies in the United States.

These changes were largely lauded by the public, still reeling from the horrors of 9/11, and possibly more so than any other urban area in the United States. They were united in a sense of shared vulnerability—be it through working in high-rise buildings whose vulnerabilities were so vividly demonstrated on 9/11 (and earlier in the 1993 World Trade Center attack)—or through their common reliance on subways, buses, trains, tunnels, and bridges as residents or commuters making their livelihoods in Manhattan.

The effects of 9/11 on urban security reached far beyond New York City. Impelled by the imagery and media record of the response to 9/11, Congress and the administration began to debate legislative and policy proposals that would ultimately form the Department of Homeland Security, the largest reorganization of the federal bureaucracy since the unification of the Department of Defense.[1] It would send millions of dollars to state and local governments and link local emergency responders more closely to the federal government than had ever existed in modern US history. Arguably, some of the lessons of 9/11 would be heeded more faithfully in many locales across the United States than in the city itself.

Following the traumatic experience of 9/11,[2] the dyad of the public and their government—through the lens of the media—reshaped expectations and perceptions in ways that are still ongoing. These changing relationships have far-reaching effects not only on the public perception of terrorism and their perceived vulnerability, but also for law enforcement and the very constructs *freedom* and *liberty* embodied by Benjamin Franklin's oft-cited if unqualified quote from 1755: "Those who would give up essential Liberty, to purchase a little temporary Safety, deserve neither Liberty nor Safety."[3]

This chapter will argue that there are important and often overlooked material dimensions of local government management and preparedness that underlie these lofty ideals. These dimensions include such prosaic

concerns as: interagency rivalry, incident management protocols, training, communications, and sustaining the extraordinary commitments to
emergency services by the elected officials and bureaucrats made in the
haze of the smoldering ruins of the World Trade Center and Pentagon. In
addition, the very success of the NYPD and an attitude of unquestioning
acceptance by elected officials and the press after 9/11 have ironically led
to its power's being challenged both politically and legally.

In fact, the platitudes, mythmaking, and hyperbole that have come
to dominate public discourse have served in many ways to obscure and
avoid critical questions of local preparedness and policy, while creating
an unwarranted illusion of invulnerability and effectiveness. This illusion
can perpetuate the vulnerabilities that were originally set to be reduced
following 9/11.

## Nature of the Threats

Urbanized areas are faced with numerous hazards, of which terrorism is
one of great concern. In 2002, President George W. Bush's "Proposal for
Forming the Department of Homeland Security" bluntly defined the terrorism risk by stating "terrorists today can strike at any place, at any time,
and with virtually any weapon."[4] As this is being written, that assessment
is more salient today than perhaps at any time since 9/11. When we think
of threats facing urban areas, we must be comprehensive and creative.

The reality of that statement is both simple and staggering in the
myriad possibilities it raises. In the years since 9/11, concerns for cataclysmic attack scenarios involving chemical, biological, radiological, nuclear, or explosive devices or materials have remained grim scenarios that
inform worst-case preparations and plans. While these concerns have
dominated many of the post–9/11 preparations, other less exotic threats
have pushed them from the forefront of public consciousness.

The urban form itself complicates protective efforts because population, employment, and valuable building stock and infrastructure are
closely packed. The concentration of economic activity, iconic structures,
and populations is unparalleled. New York's urban region of over 20 million people is linked by an aging infrastructure and sprawling mass transit
systems.

New York City is and will remain the preeminent terror target in the
United States for several reasons. It has iconic value, representing America
across the world. It is a major port of entry for international travel, directly accessible from many nations. Its density and urban form provide

large numbers of people in many venues, including common areas such as streets, plazas, and mass transit facilities and conveyances. Perhaps equally important is the presence of multiple media outlets, assuring that events here receive global coverage in near-real-time. Since 1970, 13.1 percent of all terrorist attacks in the United States occurred in the Borough of Manhattan, with additional attacks in the metropolitan area.[5]

As an example of terrorism's impact on the city, a 2008 national survey found that New York residents had the highest percentage of respondents who indicated that they were affected by terrorism. Over 60 percent of the New Yorkers contacted indicated that they had been affected, versus less than 50 percent of Washington, DC, residents, and less than 25 percent for residents in Los Angeles or the rest of the country.[6]

The reality of securing New York City from terrorists is somewhere between extremely difficult and impossible. While we speak of terrorism, we also should distinguish between the scale of attacks. While events such as 9/11 are certainly possible, protection from such events falls primarily on the resources of the federal government in terms of their controls over immigration, travel, foreign intelligence, foreign policy, and the military.

In an urban setting such as New York City, efforts to enhance security can increase concentration of targets. In an environment that is rich in targets, protecting one target can merely displace the threat to another adjacent or less protected target. Setting up a checkpoint for screening vehicles or people can create a large concentration of vehicles or people that are themselves susceptible to attack. For example, we have seen airport attacks occur in the queues for passenger screening outside the secured areas.

Department of Homeland Security (DHS), in its assessment of terrorist attack methods, lists fourteen methods of attack, ranging from aircraft as a weapon, hostage taking, chemicals, and radiological dispersal devices to food or water contamination.[7] All are potential threats to New York City. The purpose of this chapter is not to list every method but to demonstrate that there are many—and that they range in sophistication from spur of the moment efforts by individuals to more elaborate attacks involving teams of trained and equipped personnel.

One arguable effect of the Global War on Terror is the disruption of networks that had the capacity that could plan, support, and execute complex, large-scale attacks. Of course, when assessing terror risk, we must consider the periodicity of attacks. The eight-year gap between the 1993 World Trade Center bombing and the 2001 attack indicates that adversaries' planning cycles may not coincide with US electoral calendars or agency budgets. Just because we haven't had an attack does not mean that we won't be attacked.

Assuming that terrorists are barred from access to more destructive tools, the threat may be evolving toward simpler methods. The coordinated assaults on Mumbai on November 26, 2008, demonstrated the potential for damage and loss even with conventional weapons. The evolving terror threat is moving toward use of more prosaic weapons—guns and improvised explosives—in the hands of individuals or small groups. The confluence of mental illness, terrorism, and criminally callous disregard for life has elevated mass shooting to a nearly commonplace occurrence in the United States.[8] Of course, the number of deaths due to terrorism is vastly outnumbered by firearm deaths from other causes.

Technology and integration of data and other networks on industrial supervisory control and data (SCADA) systems, and the continued integration of computer networks and communication in "routine" activities from banking to telephones has introduced added vulnerability. Despite fears of a cyberattack, those fears have not yet been fully realized, but hostile network instructions and unauthorized access are growing in frequency.

New York City, with its concentration of population in tall buildings dependent on elevators, water pumps, and other systems for support, would be extremely vulnerable to a cyberdisruption. Indeed, the city recently lost a lawsuit brought by advocates for people with disabilities following Hurricanes Irene and Sandy, in part due to the inability to evacuate and support high-rise residents stranded without electricity in the days and weeks following the storm.[9] This is particularly concerning because these were events with several days' notice—a condition unlikely to be met during an intentional attack. Such threats must be dealt with, and will place tremendous demands on emergency services to move, support, and sustain vulnerable populations. These demands on emergency response resources will occur at the same time that demand for other services will peak.

Technological advance has also helped in the prevention, detection, and response to terrorist attacks. Efforts by the NYPD such as the Lower Manhattan Security Initiative have focused on integrating video surveillance and other monitoring for the area south of Canal Street in Manhattan.[10] Smaller efforts to install, integrate, and monitor security cameras by police are underway throughout the city.

In addition, the rise of social media and interactive communication tools holds the potential to better link the public to emergency services.

Social media and widespread utilization of smart phones can enable improved awareness of needs by government, and better coordination with private and nonprofit groups, including grassroots aid organizations that have played a crucial role in assisting the public after disasters and would fulfill this role during or after a terrorist event. In many ways, these opportunities have yet to be realized but offer promise for the future.

Finally, the sheer size of the city and its emergency services permits an unprecedented marshaling of resources to prevent, respond to, and recover from an event. Such resources are unavailable in any other US city. Just as we are challenged, so are we advantaged.

## Sustainability of Homeland Security Funding

The formation of the US Department of Homeland Security was quickly followed by the rollout of grant programs conceived to help state and local response agencies build capacity for a range of capabilities and prepare for response to a terror attack of unknown origin and type. Grants were initially shoveled out of Washington with haste, responding both to pressure from elected officials to "bring home the bacon" of homeland security funding, and the legitimate need felt by local agency chiefs to shore up their capacity to respond to another 9/11, or even more dire attack.

### The Federal Funding Climate

Foisted onto public safety agencies with little capacity for grant administration, and even less capacity or interest in measuring performance, it was difficult to assess the impact of the federal funds flowing into agencies across the nation. Congress was generally eager to show that the nation was getting value for money spent, while specifically they lobbied for more funds (and not for strict accountability) for their own districts.

Nationally, as money flowed to fulfill hastily prepared local plans, public safety agencies were in a race to develop plans that would enable receipt of funding from their respective state homeland security agencies—most of which were formed shortly after the federal agency was "stood up." In short, there was an unprecedented amount of funds being pushed out of Washington via states with limited experience administering large grant programs and local agencies with short deadlines to apply for a set of new funding streams. In addition, as existing agency grants were repurposed for homeland security and once-independent programs were moved under

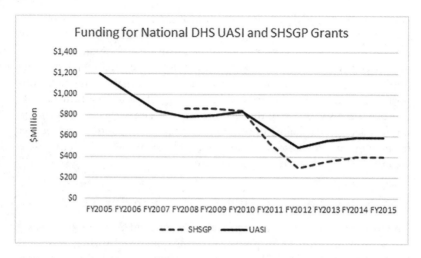

Figure 1. State Homeland Security Grant Program (FY 2008–15) and Urban Areas Security Initiative (FY 2007–15) funding streams. Credit: Charles R. Jennings

DHS, there was a transition period when reporting systems and practices were being developed from scratch or adapted from existing grant programs administered under different rules. Unsurprisingly, amid a good-faith effort by states and localities, some anecdotal horror stories of waste or misuse of funds emerged.

Following the national economic slowdown and with predictable competition for various needs, aid to state and local governments has begun to contract. Figure 1 indicates the funding for two major DHS funding streams—the State Homeland Security Grant Program (SHSGP) and the Urban Areas Security Initiative (UASI) based on DHS budgets. Both funding streams are designed to support emergency responders, and the UASI is targeted at the largest metropolitan areas in the country. The trend in funding shows clearly, on a national basis, the decline in dollars flowing to first response agencies. New York City's funding stream has not gone down as much, since several cities were eliminated from the program.

## The NYPD, Federal Funding, and Staffing

Due to its continued threat profile and a vigorous defense by its Congressional delegation, New York City has seen a more consistent flow of federal funds. The monies have supported a host of programs and helped develop many counterterrorism and preparedness programs in the city. As an example, New York City received over $118 million annually in FY2006–2008 under UASI alone.[11]

At the same time that DHS funding declined, the national recession in 2007–2008 took a toll on local agency budgets in many cities. Nationally, many first responder agencies saw layoffs and reductions in staff due to falling tax revenues during the recession.[12]

In contrast to many locales, when the NYPD reduced staff, the process was much more orderly. The NYPD actually experienced a decreasing headcount of uniformed staffing from a pre–9/11 peak of 40,300 in 2000 to its current level of less than 35,000 since 2009.[13] The NYPD continued to post declines in crime in spite of a decreased headcount due in part to the "peace dividend" from its success in reducing serious crime, and the more recent change in law enforcement policy advocated by Mayor de Blasio and his NYPD commissioners.[14]

That the NYPD confronted its most novel challenge without significantly increasing its staff was truly remarkable. Aided by abundant overtime and propped up with federal aid, the city managed a transformation in the way it approached counterterrorism and public security. This transformation would ultimately impinge on traditional intergovernmental roles in preventing terrorism.

## Federalism, Terrorism, and NYPD's Special Role

Law enforcement is a primarily local function, with an estimated 18,000 state and local police agencies protecting the United States.[15] Similarly there are approximately 30,000 fire departments and at least 21,000 emergency medical services agencies.[16] On the ground, and particularly in matters of emergency response, local emergency responders inhabit a position of primacy both in terms of their numerical dominance and their proximity to real-world events. As an example, the NYPD has more sworn officers than the Federal Bureau of Investigation (FBI), US Secret Service, US Marshals, and US Immigration and Customs Enforcement combined.[17]

Terrorism, on the contrary, is primarily a federal function, involving international relations and crossing both local domestic and international boundaries. The federal government has statutory primacy in matters of counterterrorism. Terrorist attacks are prosecuted under federal law, and the FBI is the lead agency. Before 9/11, New York did not even have a state law that addressed terrorism. From an intergovernmental perspective, local counterterrorism itself is frustrated by the cross-border activity of terrorists, who are often not residents of the locales in which they plan their attacks and may have international connections.

When the 9/11 attacks occurred, Kristin Ljungkvist observed that Mayor Rudolph Giuliani (in the last months of his term) explicitly deferred questions of the motivations and response to the attacks to the federal government.[18] The prevailing wisdom on 9/11 was that preventing terrorism is a primary responsibility of the federal government. Within New York City, all of this deference was relegated to idle academic debate within weeks. The city grew to collectively feel that the federal government—particularly the intelligence services and FBI—had let it down.

As the city came to grips with its loss, Michael Bloomberg assumed office on January 1, 2002, and appointed Ray Kelly as NYPD Commissioner for the second time. NYPD's post–9/11 transformation occurred under the watch of Mayor Bloomberg, who largely managed public safety in a hands-off style, with the NYPD securely dominant in the sphere of public safety, and with the FDNY and Office of Emergency Management playing minor supporting roles. Within months, Kelly had created a Counterterrorism Division and explicitly began to challenge the boundaries of local law enforcement's role in counterterrorism. We don't intend to retell that entire story (see Ljungkvist as an example) but will focus on those aspects that most critically bear on emergency response and public security.

The Counterterrorism Division hired analysts and interpreters to monitor global media and intelligence, as well as get a better awareness of activities among the City's diverse population. However, two vignettes are instructive to the mindset of the NYPD as the principal agency battling terrorism. The first was establishment of the International Liaison Program (ILP). The ILP is described on the Police Foundation website:

> Intelligence Officers are stationed in 11 international cities, working with law enforcement agencies to provide firsthand, in-depth analysis to New York City. The world-wide presence allows NYPD officers at the scene of a terrorist attack to provide information to the NYPD's counterterrorism command structure.

> The ILP offers an outstanding model of how public-private collaborations can impact public safety. The City of New York underwrites the personnel costs of the officers. The New York City Police Foundation, through contributions from its business, individual and

philanthropic partners provides essential travel, lodging, and office expenses that fall outside the city's budgetary lines.

Although Kelly himself admitted that the program produced no leads that thwarted a terrorist attack, there are remarks from federal law enforcement and intelligence sources that the program is ineffective.[19] The program remains in near-universal high regard among local elected officials, media, and has begrudging acquiescence by the federal government. In spite of criticisms, the program benefits from a widely held public perception that the NYPD's role is both appropriate and effective. The program has thus far continued in the de Blasio era.

## Incident Management: NYPD and FDNY

The other sentinel issue in New York post–9/11 is the city's protocol for mediating responsibility for incident management. This was illustrated most clearly by the city's efforts to implement a federal mandate for the National Incident Management System (NIMS) and the Incident Command System (ICS). NIMS/ICS were long-established procedures for dividing responsibility for managing large, complex incidents. Although they originated largely from wildfire incident management techniques originating in California in the 1970s, by 2001 they were well accepted in the fire services and emergency management communities but less so in law enforcement.

The subtext of many post–9/11 changes was the cultural clash between police and fire that led to the ruinous decision to operate separate command posts for these critical agencies during the World Trade Center event. To counter the widely held belief that dysfunction within emergency services leadership in New York City would go unchanged, the city was required to adopt national incident management protocols to assure their eligibility for homeland security funds.

The city dithered for years after 9/11 before producing its "solution." Meanwhile, the rest of the country put aside petty bickering among their public safety agencies and adopted systems consistent with or adapted directly from federal doctrine.

In a gesture demonstrating the city's bureaucratic intransigence and disdain of anything that did not come from New York City itself, the city took the long-standing federal doctrine for incident management and, in their own inimitable custom, adapted it. The changes included identification of a matrix of incident responsibility, which would assign incidents to a "lead agency." One of the key tenets of the NIMS was the concept of "unified command." Unified command was designed to be used in incidents for which no single agency had the personnel, training, equipment, and skills to mitigate an incident.[20]

The adoption of a formal incident management protocol was intended to avoid the dysfunctional quibbling and uneasy "push and shove" of negotiating responsibility for incidents. In reality, the causality and even origin of an incident can be unclear and take some time to ascertain. For example, an apparent explosion could be caused by a leak of natural gas or an explosive device. Additionally, even in the case of a natural gas leak, the leak could have been initiated by a criminal act or a mechanical defect. In reality, the clean and crisp delineations in the Citywide Incident Management System (CIMS) can dissolve in the stress of a large, rapidly unfolding event.

Nonetheless, in the case of a hazardous materials response, NYPD was designated the lead agency until such time that the incident was determined not to be the result of a terrorist or criminal act. This decision flew in the face of conventional wisdom and practice. The NYPD and FDNY are torn over competing impulses—preserve the crime scene and potential evidence, versus effecting immediate unfettered rescue and fire control. The other artifice of CIMS is that FDNY is equipped to enter a hazardous environment and would likely arrive on scene before police and in superior numbers.

CIMS remains silent on this critical question and introduces a potential for unproductive and contentious delay. Implementation of the system was largely perceived as driven by the NYPD, with the City's Office of Emergency Management thrust into the public role of "neutral arbiter." The relatively tiny, civilian Office of Emergency Management ostensibly took credit for "implementing" the system, which is like expecting the Boy Scouts to moderate a disagreement between the Army and Marines.

The FDNY vehemently opposed the proposed changes, with FDNY's Chief of Department Peter Hayden stating in 2005 that the system, as conceived, "was a recipe for disaster."[21] Mayor Bloomberg, however, adopted the new plan. The City Council, left out of the process, called for a hearing. The Bloomberg administration initially barred representatives of police or fire from testifying before council and planned to send only the commissioner of emergency management, most likely to avoid a public dispute between police and fire. After objections from council, which issued a subpoena for the appearance of the FDNY chief, the mayor's office relented. By then, the wayward fire chief was brought back on message and vowed to comply with the orders under direct threat from Mayor Bloomberg.[22]

By the time of the May 2005 City Council hearing, the issue had become a full-blown spectacle. Joining the commissioners of NYPD and FDNY were Commissioner of Emergency Management Joseph Bruno, FDNY Chief of Department Peter Hayden, union officials for the police and fire departments, and a slate of outside experts called by the council to weigh in on the controversial decision. Chief Hayden's testimony was punctuated by ovations from a crowd of firefighters in attendance and overflowing out to the streets surrounding City Hall. Council members universally praised Hayden for his courage in standing up to the administration.

Every outside expert, including Jerome Hauer, the city's first and best regarded head of emergency management, Glenn Corbett of John Jay College of Criminal Justice (9/11 reform advocate and well-known fire service author), and Jim Schwartz, fire chief from Arlington County, Virginia (who commanded the well-regarded Pentagon response on 9/11), condemned the CIMS document as not complying with the federal NIMS standard and being contrary to good practice. On the other side, a panel of police union representatives testified in support of CIMS.[23]

In spite of the raucous hearing, the Bloomberg administration pressed forward with CIMS essentially as written, laying the groundwork for smoldering resentment and delivering a decisive victory for the NYPD in a decades-long "battle of the badges."[24] The dysfunction of the 9/11 response was in some measure baked into the city's premier reform step. FDNY Chief Hayden would be gone within a year, and the City would not change the hazardous materials response protocol.

The ascendance of the NYPD and its legitimate primacy in protecting the city from terrorism marked the beginning of a period of unchecked autonomy and power under the Bloomberg administration, which took a largely "hands-off" approach to public safety, leaving the power imbalance between his powerful police commissioner and outmatched fire and emergency management commissioners to fester.

There was ample room for concern following the city's belated and inelegant adoption of CIMS. Indeed, careful watchers of the NYPD and FDNY continued to see a repeat of historical patterns of ambiguity and conflict in those rare incidents where the inability to coordinate was laid bare and exposed to public scrutiny. As an example, a window washer rescue in 2012, one of those incidents in which FDNY and NYPD had overlapping responsibility, saw FDNY cutting through a window to bring in stranded window washers as police came down the side of the building on ropes, unbeknownst to the firefighters.[25] A subsequent incident occurred in 2016 in which an armed, barricaded subject apparently set off a smoke bomb, leading to a response from the FDNY. The FDNY officer walked through police lines, past heavily armed federal and NYPD officers, and went into the house where he was promptly shot by the subject inside. Fortunately, he was not seriously wounded. Nonetheless, the incident raised serious questions about interagency coordination.[26]

## Mass Media, Risk Communication, and Public Expectations

The other critical dimension of understanding the security of New York City is the role of the media as it serves to communicate information that the public uses for understating and formulating their perceptions of risk, and how elected officials in turn react to and represent government action and capability in response to public expectations. The application of risk information, pronouncements of local government preparedness, and political dialogue are crucial to understanding New York's adaptation to the threat of terrorism and its evolution.

New York is undeniably a world media capital. Its local broadcast stations are the flagships of the industry. The standards of journalism and the healthy skepticism that once dominated the relationship between the press and public safety went into decline as media, seeking to avoid appearing callous to the horrible losses among the FDNY, Port Authority Police, and NYPD on 9/11, were restrained in their coverage of public safety. Tough questions were avoided, and as a consequence, a chance to enrich the public dialogue and hold agencies accountable was missed.

At the same time, the craft of investigative reporting was in decline in the industry. This combination of withdrawal of support for investigative journalism, public fear of terrorism, and the Bloomberg administration's unwavering support for the NYPD created a "perfect storm" for the accumulation of power and influence by the NYPD and its charismatic Commissioner, Ray Kelly. While NYPD moved ahead with a seasoned law enforcement professional at its helm, both FDNY and Office of Emergency Management were led by civilians with no uniformed experience. Joe Bruno had had an undistinguished term as fire commissioner and had taken a judgeship before being brought back to lead the critical emergency management function by Mayor Bloomberg. FDNY's Nicholas Scopetta, though well regarded as a City Hall "fixer" who led numerous agencies, had no expertise in fire or emergency services. This imbalance in aggressiveness, knowledge of the job, and professional stature further contributed to the trend, as NYPD's narrative had no counterweight within the city government.

Amid this environment of an ascending NYPD, a dynamic emerged for oversight and reportage on the city's counterterrorism efforts: first, the adoption of a "support the NYPD or risk terrorism" mindset, and second, the repetition of the "zero risk" narrative.

Commissioner Kelly and the NYPD have advanced the narrative that sixteen plots have been thwarted since 9/11. We will not further contest this assertion, although it is safe to say that there is widely divergent opinion on the matter in regard to the credibility of the plots, and NYPD's role, as expressed previously.[27]

The media, aided by the rhetoric of elected officials, have actively cultivated this illusion of safety. Law enforcement stokes this narrative to acquire and increase the resources needed to protect the public. Elected officials are complicit by both offering lip service to law enforcement's effort and promoting their own roles in assuring public safety. Nowhere is the invincibility or "zero risk" narrative more evident than in the contention by Commissioner Kelly, originally made in a *60 Minutes* interview in 2011, that the NYPD had the wherewithal to shoot down an aircraft (on authority of Mayor Bloomberg) threatening the city.[28]

There have been notable cracks in the city's armor of invincibility. Notable security lapses—such as the prank spray painting of the Brooklyn Bridge in 2012, under supposed constant surveillance—were major embarrassments to the NYPD.[29] In 2014, in an apparent rogue art project, the two American flags that fly atop the Brooklyn Bridge were replaced with white flags.[30] Most seriously, the origins of a bomb placed in the heart of Times Square, one of the most heavily surveilled and patrolled locales in the city, remains unsolved after seven years.[31] Of course, the city's closest brush with a terror plot that moved beyond the planning stage occurred on May 1, 2010, when an improvised explosive device left in a parked car failed to detonate. That incident was originally reported as a car fire. Alerted by street vendors, the responding police and firefighters recognized the suspicious nature of the incident and withdrew.[32] Had the device been successful, it would have detonated, likely resulting in numerous casualties.

The role of the press in creating this chasm between rhetoric and reality is summarized by James Fallows, who spells out the hazards of building up the capability and likelihood of terrorist acts:

Let's start with the First Rule of Terrorism, which this era's attackers either know instinctively or have learned. That rule is: The purpose of terrorism is not to kill or maim or destroy. For the attackers, such crimes are merely tactics, on the way to a different goal, which is *to terrorize*. The strategic ambition is to use attacks and atrocities to change people's emotions and arouse their fears. The aim is to make strong societies feel desperate and helpless, and to make objectively very small threats seem subjectively very large.[33]

Some researchers argue that terrorism receives disproportionate attention, but there is room for debate and considerable uncertainty. The reality of limited resources requires that difficult choices be made on investments in security.[34]

In this sense, the twenty-four-hour news cycle and the continuous repetition of minimal facts known about an attack, attempted attack, or even an averted attack tend to sensationalize and enhance the perception of risk for many members of the public. Reacting in part to the implicit logic that the government is extraordinarily effective in detecting and disrupting terror plots, media tend to imbue attackers with supreme rationality, ability, and guile. For example, a casual search of headlines following the 2015 Paris terror attacks finds reference to the leader as "mastermind" in US media. Media critics have noted the cooperation of journalists both in building up Osama bin Laden from criminal to global mastermind and the media's complicity in supporting the government's "wartime" narrative.[35]

Further, the release and constant repeating of information about potential attacks, especially those foiled in their early stages, can feed into the cycle of fear that drives the public to accept any measure that promises to reduce perceived risk. As such, leaking details of planned attacks, particularly if done for political gain, can be disingenuous. As described by Gabe Mythen and Sandra Walklate, "It is probable that each exposure of a 'terrorist plot' serves to ratchet up levels of public concern about terrorism."[36] Rather than being used to drum up support or justify particular policies or programs, risk information can be purposefully utilized to help the public better prepare and to assure rather than to alarm.[37]

For examples of the tension between "cheerleading" coverage and responsible and helpful media, Andrea Dunkin in 2004 explicitly acknowledged the symbolic appropriation of first responders as heroes and the rallying point for the nation following 9/11. The centrality of first responders to the rallying of the nation made it more challenging to offer critical assessments of their performance. As an example of exemplary journalism, Dunkin cites Jim Dwyer and Kevin Flynn's 2005 book *102 Minutes: The Unforgettable Story of the Fight to Survive Inside the Twin Towers,* which documented the heroism but candidly identified shortcomings and areas for improvement, ultimately helping make the city safer.[38]

## Opportunities for Realism and Lessons for the Future

Criticisms in this chapter are not intended to besmirch the work of the police officers, EMS workers, firefighters, and emergency managers who have labored mightily since 9/11 to keep New York City safe and make it better prepared for and less susceptible to attack. The NYPD's stance following 9/11, particularly its decision to launch a major counterterrorism effort, undoubtedly helped contribute to a perception of a greatly hardened city, which likely dampened the enthusiasm of prospective attackers. It also helped the agency meaningfully interact with the global flow of information and intelligence to maintain awareness and foster adaptation to changing circumstances. Similarly, I write with appreciation of the tremendous strides made in advancing the capacity of emergency response organizations within New York City since 9/11.

With the election of Bill de Blasio in 2014 and replacement of the principals in charge of New York City's primary response agencies—police, fire, and emergency management—we can hope that the long-standing patterns of competition will continue to evolve toward a more collaborative, multidisciplinary approach to emergency response. Initial signs, such as the formation of the Critical Response Command by the NYPD, point to a more sustainable pattern of deploying personnel, while increasing capability to react to the emergent threat of multiple assailants with firearms and small explosive devices.[39] We hope that the FDNY will be closely integrated into the City's efforts to respond to novel threats.[40]

For meaningful change to come, the traditional bluster of invincibility and unquestioning attitudes of elected officials and the public must be aided by a more thorough and critical journalism that investigates claims of preparedness and the carefully orchestrated exercises done both to reassure the public and to sustain the narrative of a reformed emergency response system. Stage-managed events are dutifully presented to the public, while little effort is invested in digging beneath the surface to better test the city's readiness.

Such scrutiny and oversight of day-to-day activities of emergency services are critical. The connection between the mundane world that has included shootings, stranded window washers, fires, and response times is not only necessary but also essential. Monitoring performance at these "everyday' incidents is essential to assuring the city's sophisticated efforts to prevent, prepare for, respond to, and ultimately recover from not just terrorism, but all disasters. The dividend of this robust capability will reap benefits during disasters that will likely come from nature, technological failure, as well as intentional acts, regardless of motivation.

Although one can question how seriously some people took the lessons of 9/11, the event demonstrated the highly interdependent nature of response to various kinds of emergencies in an urban context. Similarly, Hurricane Sandy crossed boundaries between neat conceptions of agency roles, revealing shortcomings in the city's preparation and execution of plans for dealing with large-scale disaster events. Creating an integrated response to large-scale events remains a challenge for New York.

Indeed, analyses of the response to the 9/11 attack in New York make it evident that a cross-disciplinary analysis of response to emergencies was warranted. Looking from the single-agency perspective that still dominates official thinking misses opportunities to identify crosscutting areas for improvement. Doing so would permit agencies to develop processes that avoid contentious encounters following a significant event.[41] And perhaps most important, these reviews should be shared with the public.

When glaring problems *are* identified, the need for objective, independent review is obvious, but seldom certain. Following a recent "active shooter" scare at JFK Airport, thousands of patrons reported hours of uncertainty and fear as they received conflicting instructions. The event was marked by communication problems, uncertainty, and finger pointing by multiple agencies.[42] Such incidents raise deep questions about the readiness of the city's response system. Unfortunately, the urgent calls for inquiry are defused by a flurry of pronouncements and half-promises for reviews that seldom come to light or persist across news cycles. Even when "solutions" are promised, elected officials and the media seldom follow up to see if changes were implemented and sustained.

Rather than accept an honest view of safety and mentally preparing for the real but risk-informed eventuality of an attack, we have instead been seduced by a comforting—but ultimately hollow—promise of safety in the face of well-intended but clearly inadequate efforts by government to manage the risk in the face of insurmountable odds. Therefore, the time has come for a more transparent, honest dialogue between government, elected officials, and the public. Only then can we begin to assess the investments in homeland security and weigh them against the real costs they impose, not only in governmental budgets but also in their impact on the way of life and values we cherish as New Yorkers.

## Conclusion

On a political level, the election of Bill de Blasio in 2014, who swept into City Hall on a platform of greater police accountability and control, was in part a reaction to Michael Bloomberg. Mayor Bloomberg had ceded his role in overseeing and restraining the NYPD's impulses for greater authority and power to pursue not only their unquestioned agenda for counterterrorism and civil protection from foreign terror, but their on-going pursuit of ever-lower crime statistics.[43] This agenda was fulfilled in no small measure through constitutionally suspect exercise of police power on politically weak segments of the city's population.[44]

The contribution of the post–9/11 confluence of homeland security and sustained inattention of political oversight through over a decade of Mayoral administrations must surely be listed as a contributing factor. Most critically, as was demonstrated earlier, the fortress NYPD cemented its relative power over emergency response and management in the City with adoption of the Citywide Incident Management System (CIMS). Despite objections raised in its hasty and controversial adoption, it continues to this day. Meaningful adjustment or study of this policy's effects has been largely absent. If this political and bureaucratic acquiescence has deferred a reckoning of the vulnerability that was so brutally and plainly exposed on 9/11 remains to be seen. The NYPD's prestige and its perceived success in both continuing to lower crime and fight terrorism ironically contributed to a "hands-off" attitude by elected officials.

The crescendo of community rancor and concern erupted once the Bloomberg administration was out of power. Rather than an orderly and incremental self-correction moderated by engagement with the public and elected officials, numerous legislative reforms were imposed on the department by a skeptical City Council and de Blasio administration, buttressed by court rulings.

Since 9/11, the city's public safety landscape has changed in many positive ways. However, the combination of limited oversight and bureaucratic intransigence have not only resulted in diminished autonomy of the NYPD but also sowed the seeds for uncertainty in response to complex future threats that New York City will undoubtedly face.

### Notes

1. Bush, 2002.
2. See, for example, Strozier, 2011.

3. Eugene Volokh, "Liberty, Safety, and Benjamin Franklin," *Washington Post*, November 11, 2014; Wittes, 2011.

4. Bush, 2002.

5. LaFree and Bersani, 2012, 16.

6. Kano, Wood, Mileti, and Bourque, 2008, 70.

7. US Department of Homeland Security, 2008.

8. Cohen, Azrael, and Miller, 2014.

9. Marc Santora and Benjamin Weiser, "Court Says New York Neglected Disabled in Emergencies," *New York Times*, November 7, 2013.

10. NYPD, "Counterterrorism Units."

11. Office of Inspector General, 2011, 24.

12. Shaila Dewan and Motoko Rich, "Public Workers Face New Rash of Layoffs, Hurting Recovery," *New York Times,* June 19, 2012.

13. O'Brien, 2015.

14. NYPD, "Crime."

15. Reaves, 2011.

16. Haynes and Stein, 2014, 16; National Highway Traffic Safety Administration, 2014.

17. Reaves, 2012.

18. Ljungkvist, 2016, 77.

19. Cushing, 2014; Jeff Stein, "NYPD Intelligence Detectives Go Their Own Way," *Washington Post*, November 11, 2010.

20. Federal Emergency Management Agency, 2009, 49.

21. Michelle O'Donnell, "City Hall Limits Testimony on Emergency Protocols," *New York Times*, April 28, 2005.

22. Stephanie Gaskell, "Mayor Slaps down FDNY Rebel over 9/11 Rules," *New York Post*, May 11, 2005.

23. New York City Council, 2005.

24. Buntin, 2005.

25. Al Baker, "17 Floors Up, Rescues of 3 Shows Clash of Agencies," *New York Times,* April 13, 2016.

26. Maura Grunlund, "Smoke, Gunfire, and Bloodshed: Inside the Mariner's Harbor Standoff," *Staten Island Advance*, August 14, 2015.

27. Elliott, 2012.

28. Colvin, 2011.

29. Marc Morales, "Brooklyn Bridge Defaced by Vandals in First Time Since Anti-Guiliani Scrawl in 1998," *New York Daily News*, June 29, 2012.

30. Vivian Yee, "A Brooklyn Bridge Mystery: Who Raised the White Flags?" *New York Times*, July 22, 2014.

31. Marc Santora and Michael Schwirtz, "F.B.I. Cites 'Persons of Interest' in 2008 Times Square Bomb Case," *New York Times*, April 15, 2015.

32. NYPD, "Terrorist Plots Targeting New York City."

33. Fallows, 2015.

34. Mueller, 2004; Stewart and Mueller, 2014; Aven, 2015.

35. Bonner, 2011.

36. Mythen and Walklate, 2008; see also Nellis and Savage, 2012.

37. Fischoff, 2011.

38. Andrea Dunkin, "Review Essay: Journalism after 9/11," *Newark Metro*, September 2006.

39. City of New York, 2015.

40. Pfeiffer, 2013.

41. Jennings, 2009.

42. Wallace-Wells, 2016.

43. Eterno and Silverman, 2012.

44. *Floyd et al v. City of New York*, 959 F. Supp. 2d 540l; Apuzzo, 2013.

## References

Apuzzo, Matt. *Enemies Within: Inside the NYPD's Secret Spying Unit and Bin Laden's Final Plot Against America*. New York: Touchstone Books, 2013.

Aven, Terje. "On the Allegations That Small Risks Are Treated Out of Proportion to Their Importance." *Reliability Engineering and System Safety* 140 (2015): 116–121.

Bonner, James. "The Media and 9/11: How We Did." *The Atlantic*, September 9, 2011.

Buntin, John. "Battle of the Badges." *Governing Magazine*, September 2005.

Bush, George W. "Proposal to Create the Department of Homeland Security." White House, Washington, DC, June 2002. https://goo.gl/5zpMv8.

City of New York. "Transcript: Mayor de Blasio and Commissioner Bratton Announce First Deployment of NYPD's New Critical Response Command." November 16, 2015. https://goo.gl/pZbb9f.

Cohen, Amy P., Deborah Azrael, and Matthew Miller. "Rate of Mass Shootings Has Tripled Since 2011, Harvard Study Shows." *Mother Jones*, October 15, 2014.

Colvin, Jill. "Order to Shoot Down Planes Would Come From Mayor, Kelly Says." *DNAinfo* (New York), October 7, 2011. https://goo.gl/kFtphC.

Cushing, Tim. "Posting of NYPD Officers Around the World Found to Be a Waste, Embarrassment." *Techdirt*, January 10, 2014. https://goo.gl/qT5Kf6.

Elliott, Justin. "Fact-Check: How the NYPD Overstated Its Counterterrorism Record." *ProPublica*, July 10, 2012. https://goo.gl/fRdDah.

Eterno, John A., and Eli Silverman. *The Crime Numbers Game: Management by Manipulation*. Boca Raton, FL: CRC Press, 2012.

Fallows, James. "CNN Shares Responsibility for the Fear-Mongering of the GOP Debate." *The Atlantic*, December 16, 2015.

Federal Emergency Management Agency. "National Incident Management System." Washington, DC, December 2009. https://goo.gl/5JAGuJ.

Fischoff, Baruch. "Communicating About the Risks of Terrorism (or Anything Else)." *American Psychologist* 66, no. 6 (September 2011): 520–531.

Haynes, Hilton, and Gary Stein. "U.S. Fire Department Profile, 2013." National Fire Protection Association, November 2014.

Jennings, Charles R. "Working Paper 09-01: Concept for Implementation of a Lessons Learned Capability for Presidentially-Declared Disasters." Christian Regenhard Center for Emergency Response Studies, New York, 2009. https://goo.gl/fjx2wj.

Kano, Megumi, Michele M. Wood, Dennis S. Mileti, and Linda B. Bourque. "Public Response to Terrorism: Findings from the National Survey of Disaster Experiences and Preparedness." The Southern California Injury Prevention Research Center and The Center for Public Health and Disasters, University of California Los Angeles, School of Public Health, Los Angeles, November 12, 2008.

LaFree, Gary, and Bianca Bersani. "Hot Spots of Terrorism and Other Crimes in the United States, 1970 to 2008." National Consortium for the Study of Terrorism and Responses to Terrorism, College Park, MD, January 31, 2012. https://goo.gl/XTouXq.

Leavitt, Leonard. "Banking on Banks." *NYPD Confidential*, April 11, 2016.

Ljungkvist, Kristin. *The Global City 2.0: From Strategic Site to Global Actor.* New York: Routledge, 2016.

Mueller, John. "A False Sense of Insecurity? How Does the Risk of Terrorism Measure up against Everyday Dangers?" *Regulation* 27, no. 3 (2004): 42–46.

Mythen, Gabe, and Sandra Walklate. "Terrorism, Risk, and International Security: The Perils of Asking 'What If?'" *Security Dialogue* 39, no. 2–3 (April 2008): 221–242.

National Highway Traffic Safety Administration. "EMS Data is Important." *Safety in Numbers Newsletter,* May 2014. https://goo.gl/2mHWTc.

Nellis, Ashley Marie, and Joanne Savage. "Does Watching the News Affect Fear of Terrorism? The Importance of Media Exposure on Terrorism and Fear." *Crime and Delinquency* 58, no. 5 (2012): 748–768.

New York City Council. "Transcripts of the Minutes of the May 9, 2005 Hearing of the Committee on Fire and Criminal Justice Services Jointly with the Committee on Public Safety." May 9, 2005.

New York City Police Department. "Counterterrorism Units." February 16, 2016. https://goo.gl/hqdPWB.

———. "Crime." February 16, 2016.

———. "Terrorist Plots Targeting New York City."

O'Brien, Bernard. "Uniformly Overbudget: Tracing Police Overtime Spending and Staffing Since 1996." New York City Independent Budget Office, May 2015.

Office of the Inspector General. "OIG-11-30: The State of New York's Management of State Homeland Security Program and Urban Areas

Security Initiative Grants Awarded During Fiscal Years 2006 through 2008."
US Department of Homeland Security, Washington, DC, January 2011.
https://goo.gl/FLkjvY.

Pfeiffer, Joseph W. "Fire as a Weapon in Terrorist Attacks." *Combating Terrorism Center Sentinel*, July 23, 2013. https://goo.gl/ErWjfY.

Reaves, Brian J. "Census of State and Local Law Enforcement Agencies, 2008."
US Department of Justice, Bureau of Justice Statistics, 2011. https://goo.gl/5uWm2u.

———. "Federal Law Enforcement Officers, 2008." US Department of Justice, Bureau of Justice Statistics, 2012. https://goo.gl/GeanPG.

Stewart, Mark G., and John Mueller. "Cost-Benefit Analysis of Airport Security: Are Airports Too Safe?" *Journal of Air Transport Management*, 35 (2014): 19–28.

Strozier, Charles. *Until the Fires Stopped Burning: 9/11 and New York City in the Words and Experiences of Survivors and Witnesses*. New York: Columbia University Press, 2011.

US Department of Homeland Security. "Potential Terrorist Attack Methods Joint Special Assessment." Washington, DC, April 23, 2008. https://goo.gl/nPMMqJ.

Wallace-Wells, David. "Scenes from the Terrifying, Already Forgotten JFK Airport Shooting that Wasn't." *New York Magazine*, August 2016.

Wittes, Benjamin. "Against a Crude Balance: Platform Security and the Hostile Symbiosis Between Liberty and Security." Harvard Law School/Brookings Institution Project on Law and Security, Boston, MA, September 21, 2011. https://goo.gl/VLeShL.

# Managing Fire Emergencies in Tall Buildings
## Design Innovations in the Wake of 9/11

Norman Groner

Imagine that you are on the fiftieth floor of a tall office building and that the fire alarm begins to sound. People look around at each other, wondering whether this could be a real emergency, or more likely, a fire drill or alarm system malfunction. But it is a lot of trouble to take action when everyone is working and meeting, so people understandably wait until they have better information. A few minutes later, someone looks out the window and sees that the fire department has arrived. Someone calls down to the security desk in the lobby, but no one answers. Some occupants decide that they should leave and discover that the elevator is still working, and an argument ensues about whether it can be safely used. After all, fifty flights of stairs is a very long way to walk.

Then there is a faint smell of smoke and a light haze. Most people decide that they should leave, but the stairs are crowded and they have to queue to enter. Other people decide to wait longer because, even if they can enter the stairs, they know that their physical condition would likely result in injury by taking such an arduous journey. The haze thickens, the acrid smell worsens, and eyes start to sting and water. People are getting very scared. There's no obvious action that will ensure safety.

People naturally tend to pay little thought to highly remote risks, and prior to the 9/11 World Trade Center (WTC) attacks, there was little reason to worry about this type of scenario. But the possibility became vividly apparent after 9/11. This chapter examines the technological and regulatory reactions following 9/11 that have improved the safety in tall buildings, with a particular focus on using elevators to evacuate tall buildings, even during a fire emergency. Because timely escape from tall building is difficult, these structures are inherently vulnerable to attacks and other disasters.

Changes in safety practices typically follow tragic events, so it comes as no surprise that tall building safety was scrutinized extensively following the World Trade Center attacks. In this chapter we review progress in helping people find safety when tall buildings are subjected to fires and other perils. In particular, New York City has been the focus of many of the proposed and realized changes. Of all the innovations, perhaps the use of elevators during fire emergencies is the most startling and promising.

Despite improvements in code requirements following the WTC attacks, however, technological changes are not always positive. Rather, many changes are primarily motivated by reducing the costs of construction. In the last decade, a rash of facade fires in tall buildings culminated in the tragic fire at the Grenfell Tower in London, for example, resulting in the deaths of seventy-one persons. Thus, vigilance in testing and regulating technological innovations remains crucial.

## Working and Living in Tall Buildings: Perceptions of Safety

People remained uncomfortable after the WTC attacks at working in tall buildings—at least for a while. Some were scared. Some were traumatized. News reporters interviewed people who said that they had to move from the city and would never work or live in a high-rise building again. Indeed, New Yorkers remained nervous at least a decade following September 11 as revealed by a modestly sized earthquake (magnitude 5.8), centered in Virginia, that was easily noticeable in tall buildings in Manhattan. Although occupants of modern building are likely to be safer remaining inside to avoid debris falling from the building's exterior, many people self-evacuated from buildings[1] presumably without instructions from building management. Regardless, the fear of working and living in tall buildings soon subsided for most New Yorkers, at least among persons not so immediately affected by the disaster.[2]

Downtown Manhattan, the site of the WTC attacks, has been undergoing a boom and high-rise buildings are vigorously sprouting throughout the city. By August 2010, there were 5,912 completed high-rises in the city, and as of November 2017, New York City has 257 buildings rising at least 492 feet (150 m) in height, with 36 more under construction. Downtown Manhattan is now a fashionable place to live and work, and it has numerous new high-rise residential towers with associated restaurants, bars, and shopping.

The unabated construction of very tall buildings is predicted to continue, with new construction techniques and technologies enabling improved energy efficiency and lower construction costs.[3] Thus, high-rise buildings remain a fixture in New York City and whatever fears resulting from the WTC attacks have been transient.

## Tall Buildings: Safe or Dangerous?

Are people safer in tall buildings than before 9/11? The answer is mostly "yes," at least for routine emergencies. However, because terrorist strikes against tall buildings can cause far more destruction than routine emergencies, terror attacks remain a significant threat.

It seems contradictory to state that high-rise buildings are both unusually safe and unusually dangerous environments. Tall buildings are unusually dangerous in that the geometry dictates that occupants must descend long distances to leave the building—a time-consuming and physically demanding task. Further, the stairs are of limited number and only have a limited capacity. Codes do not require that the stairs are large enough for all the occupants to leave the building at the same time.

That said, tall buildings are unusually safe. They are constructed to meet fire and building codes that are more stringent than those mandated for other buildings used for the same purposes. Removing data from the WTC attacks, the overall record for fire casualties in tall buildings has been very low. Most people (approximately 80 percent) who die in fires die in their own homes. And most of those fatalities occurred in buildings with much less stringent code requirements than residential high-rise structures.

Because these data are restricted to fires and not to terrorist attacks per se, how safe are people in high-rise building as opposed to other types of structures in such events? Because there isn't much data from real terrorist incidents, fire safety experts rely on hypothetical scenarios to evaluate safety. Despite the good record of safety, there is no denying the risk from acts of terrorism. Fortunately, new construction code changes are being implemented that clearly improve the likelihood that occupants will be relatively safer in high buildings even in the event of another intentional act of terrorism.

## Fire Safety: Comparing High-Rise and Other Buildings

As stated above, excluding the WTC attacks on 9/11, high-rise buildings have a better record of fire safety than shorter buildings used for the same purposes. According to John Hall, this superior safety record is probably attributable to the greater prevalence of sprinkler systems and fire-resistive construction in high-rise buildings.[4] It is important to note that the common practice is to "grandfather" existing buildings; they are not required to increase the level of fire safety to meet the requirement of codes adopted after their construction.

As an example, a 2003 fire in a Chicago office building killed six persons. In addition to operational errors by building and fire department personnel, these deaths were largely attributable to the failure to retrofit high-rise buildings with sprinkler systems and the removal of locks preventing reentry from exit stairs. Following this fire, Chicago required building owners to retrofit high-rise commercial buildings to prevent similar tragedies.

The vulnerability of high-rise buildings requires an ongoing effort to require the installation of sprinkler systems in older tall buildings, an effort that has accelerated following 9/11. New York City and most large cities in the United States require sprinkler system retrofits of high-rise office buildings, although there is generally an extended time frame to full compliance.

Outside of the United States, the 2017 multifatality fire at the Grenfell Tower in London is notable for its rapidly propagating fire along the building's exterior. However, the fire is equally attributable to the lack of a sprinkler system that allowed the fire to grow large enough to ignite the flammable exterior cladding.

## Safety Code Changes after 9/11

After 9/11, there have been changes in the code, design, and policies for tall buildings to foster safety.

### Writing New Safety Codes

The National Institute of Standards and Technology (NIST), a federal agency, investigated the collapse of the Twin Towers following the WTC center attacks and issued a report recommending code changes.[5] Before the recommendations could take effect, they required the consideration of committees charged with modifying model codes. In the United States, this nongovernmental function is fulfilled by two organizations that write the model fire and building codes: the International Code Council (ICC) and the National Fire Protection Association (NFPA). The International Code Council is responsible for writing the International Building Code and the International Fire Code. The National Fire Protection Association is responsible for the Life Safety Code, the Uniform Fire Code, and the Uniform Building Code.

Both of the model code writing organizations responded by establishing committees to make recommendations in response to 9/11. The ICC established an ad hoc Committee on Terrorism-Resistant Buildings; the NFPA established a High-Rise Building Safety Advisory Committee. Even before the code writing organizations took action, New York City convened a similar task force focusing on the city's requirements for high-rise buildings.

The process for rewriting and adopting codes is lengthy. Even after rewriting model codes, changes do not have the force of law until regulatory authorities adopt the updated editions of the model codes. The process also takes time—model codes are typically revised only once every three years, and further delays that can add years occur while waiting for governments to formally adopt and sometimes modify the model codes. Consequently, the lack of agility in improving codes has been frustrating. Indeed, it has taken a decade before many of the recommended code changes after the WTC attacks have been adopted. Even then, the more stringent requirements apply only to new construction.

*Building Code Changes Implemented after 9/11*

The International Building Code (IBC) is the most prominently adopted code in the United States. The following changes to the IBC have been made as a result of 9/11,[6] shown in Table 1.

The following sections highlight five of these post–9/11 code changes: (1) elimination of scissor stairs, (2) self-luminous exit pathways, (3) third stairways in building over 420 feet, (4) emergency evacuation elevators, and (5) fire service access elevators.

**1. Elimination of scissor stairs.** Building codes are written in an attempt to trade off concerns about safety with concerns about construction cost and operational profitability. The key to operational profitability is the amount of space that can be rented to tenants. Scissor stairs save space by placing two stairs in the same enclosure. Although they usually have remote entrances as required by codes, and they are often separated only by fire or smoke resistant partitions, these stairs are vulnerable to explosions that can destroy the partitions, rendering both stairs unusable.

In the World Trade Center towers, stairs were enclosed in the central core of the building and were mostly destroyed by the impact of the

Table 1. Building Code Changes in the International Building Code as a Result of the World Trade Center Attacks

| | |
|---|---|
| A higher standard for fire resistance in high-rise buildings more than 420 feet tall | The quality and thickness of fire resistant materials used to protect structural elements of the WTC towers was thought to have contributed to the rapid collapse of the buildings |
| More robust fireproofing for buildings more than 75 feet tall | Better fireproofing is less likely to be dislodged by impacts and explosions |
| Shafts enclosing elevators and exit stairways are now required to have impact-resistant walls | Impact-resistant walls are less likely fail in the face of explosions from terrorist and other events |
| Self-luminous exit pathway markings in all exit stairways | New photoluminescent paints and tapes will provide a lighted pathway when both the primary and secondary lighting fail |
| Improved radio coverage systems within the building | Improved communications systems will allow emergency personnel to better communicate within the building and with emergency staff outside the building |
| Elevators are required in high-rise buildings more than 120 feet tall | Elevators ensure that firefighters can get to and fight fires without walking up from the ground floor with heavy equipment, although it is unlikely that building would be constructed without such elevators anyway |
| An additional stairway for high-rises is now required for commercial buildings more than 420 feet tall | In very tall buildings, the larger numbers of occupants and the very long times required to descend might cause overcrowding of stairs |
| In lieu of the additional stairway in very tall buildings, an option to provide enhanced occupant-use elevators | Emergency occupant evacuation elevators can be used by the building occupants to speed the overall evacuation times for buildings and enable self-evacuation by occupants who cannot use stairs |

# Scissor Stairs:
# Origins, Development and Contemporary Use

**Samir Mokashi, Principal, Evergreen Engineering**

Scissor stairs have been shaping the skyline of British Columbia's burgeoning urban development and are now making spotted appearances along Portland's Willamette River. Heralded by architects and developers as a sleek way to maximize office and residential design, the scissor stair possesses an undeniable attraction. This unique stair design is not without its drawbacks however, and may not be the right fit for buildings with large floorplates.

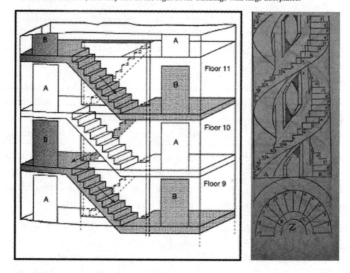

The scissor stair design is commonly known as a set of two intertwined stairs located within one stairwell enclosure. Two adjacent flights connect the same floors in opposite direction, crossing each other like a scissor, hence the name. In enclosed scissor stairs it is possible for two people to climb or descend simultaneously without ever having to meet each other. A variation of the straight scissor stair has two circular stairs winding around to form a double helix. An open version of the double helix stairs is seen in the Vatican museum. This ornate set of intertwined stairs has enthralled visitors for centuries.

Figure 1. Scissor stairs eliminated because of inadequate separation.

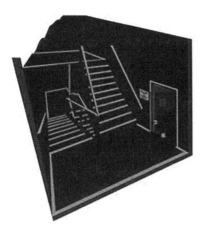

Figure 2. Photoluminescent stairway marking show exit path in the dark. Credit: EverGlo NA, Inc.

airplanes. This vulnerability became salient after the attacks because any well-placed explosive devise placed in a terrorist attack could potentially destroy all exit stairs. As a result, the codes prohibit scissor-types stairs for new construction.

2. **Self-luminous exit pathways.** Evacuations in tall buildings can take hours. Such a prolonged evacuation can exhaust backup power supplies that illuminate exit stairs and pathways, leaving means of egress dark and very slow to navigate. This problem was clearly revealed following the bombing of the WTC tower in 1993. Occupants complained about the great difficulties of evacuating in dark stairs. New technologies in photoluminescent tapes and paints have enabled marking that can remain visible for several hours. Such illumination has become widely mandated by building codes.

3. **Third stairways in building over 420 feet high.** Generally, codes do not require additional stairs as buildings grow taller. The logic is that evacuations are phased, meaning that the entire occupant load will not try to access the stairs at the same time, thereby avoiding a level of crowding that slows occupants as they descend. However, this logic is less valid as buildings increase in height. In any larger-scale emergencies, the additional numbers of occupants and the prolonged times needed to descend stairs may cause unacceptable levels of congestion. In addition, firefighters are likely to be using one of the stairs to ascend to the fire zone, thereby effectively halving the capacity of the stairs. As a result, code

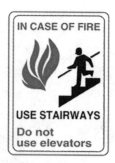

Figure 3. Sign indicating that use of the elevator is prohibited during fire emergencies.

changes, based on NIST recommendations, have been changed to require a third stairway for new buildings over 420 square feet. Because residential buildings have far fewer occupants than commercial buildings, they are exempt from the third-stairway requirement.

As noted, codes developed after 9/11 allow emergency occupant evacuation elevators to substitute for the third stairs in very tall buildings. Because elevators are always required to move building occupants in high-rise buildings, the belief is that the added expense of the upgraded fire-safe elevators can be more than offset by the added leasable floor area, at least in the long run. The features of such upgraded elevators systems are covered in the next section.

4. **Emergency occupant evacuation elevators.** The most revolutionary change in tall building egress since 9/11 is the design of "Occupant Evacuation Operation" (OEO) elevators that can be used during fire emergencies. An estimated two hundred occupants in WTC 1 and WTC 2 died in elevators on 9/11, although occupants trapped in elevators above the floors struck by the airplanes would likely have perished regardless.[7] Despite their hazards, the investigation of the WTC tower evacuations revealed that many lives were saved because elevators speeded the vertical travel of building occupants. NIST reported that "at least 18 percent of the survivors from WTC 2 [the second tower struck] reported using the elevators for at least part of their evacuation."[8]

We are all familiar with signs posted by elevators that prohibit their use during fires—and with good reason. Several deaths during high-rise fires in the 1990s highlight the hazards of their use. Heat-sensitive call buttons caused a few elevators to travel to floors with fires and open their doors. Sensors that prevent doors from closing on people entering and leaving elevators have been activated by smoke preventing the doors from closing. In some instances, persons trapped in stalled elevators lost their lives during fires.

Several design features in the current generation of elevators are intended to prevent their use during fires. The presence of smoke in elevator shafts or lobbies will cause elevators to automatically travel to the lowest safe floor where they remain inoperable with the doors open. When elevator use is evaluated as safe enough, firefighters use special keys to rescue endangered occupants and to avoid a slow and arduous climb up stairs. However, the use of elevators during a fire has inherent risk, and firefighters are reluctant to use them unless their safe use can be assessed and assured.

In recent years, there has been rapid research and development to add a new emergency operational mode for elevators that would evacuate people in order of vulnerability. Elevator lobbies and shaft ways are protected from smoke using fire-rated enclosures and pressurization. By protecting lobbies and elevators from smoke, elevators are likely to be available to evacuate people for the duration of most fire emergencies.

The large numbers of occupants who survived the WTC attacks because they used elevators gave impetus to a renewed interest in the design of elevators that could be safely used during fire emergencies. Initial research had started in the early 1990s but had languished until after 9/11. Conferences on the topic were held in the early 1990s.[9] Since that time, studies that model the speed at which buildings can be fully evacuated indicated that a tall building can be emptied in half the time it takes when express elevator service is combined with stairs. However, there was a lack of interest at the time because of the generally good safety record for tall buildings, the likely expense involved in installing elevators protected from fires, and opposition from fire departments based on their customary wariness that elevators could ever be safely used by civilians during fires.

The American Society for Mechanical Engineers organized a committee in 2005 charged with devising regulatory requirements for elevators that can be used to evacuate building occupants during fire emergencies. The resulting revisions to the Safety Code for Elevators and Escalators (ASME A17.1) specified requirements for Emergency Occupant Elevators included the following features:

The lobbies and shafts for elevators are enclosed in fire and smoke resistant barriers.
Signage is posted explaining their use during emergencies.
Elevators are protected against water that may be used during fire suppression.

Elevator lobbies are equipped with two-way communications to the fire command center, typically located in the building lobby.

Direct access to exit stairs is provided from elevator lobbies.

Software enables elevators to make express trips between floors being evacuated and the ground level.

Obstacles to using modified elevators are not primarily technological, however.[10] The most difficult issues are operational and concern who controls and who uses these protected elevators. They raise a number of important procedural and behavioral questions:

Will occupants willingly use the elevators, given the nearly universal prohibition on their use during fires? The central problem is trust, not habit. Because these will be new and special buildings, occupants will not have difficulty differentiating them from other buildings where elevators cannot be used. Trust in the technology, however, is probably the primary challenge to using protected elevators by both firefighters and occupants. Education and training are clearly required. It seems likely that occupants who can otherwise use stairs will need to understand the safeguards protecting the elevators. Persons who cannot negotiate any stairs due to mobility impairments may seem to have little choice, but even here, they will need enough confidence in the technology to leave locations that seem, at least for the time being, relatively safe. Floor wardens may be required to reassure occupants that the elevators can be safely used during an emergency.

Would people who cannot use stairs at all take priority, or would the elevators be used by any and all occupants? The idea of using elevators to evacuate buildings originated in the early 1990s with an interest in providing persons with disabilities as low a level of risk as persons who are able to descend stairs. In more recent years, evacuation models indicated that the use of elevators by any occupants who are immediately endangered by a fire improves overall safety because it enabled a more rapid evacuation of all building occupants.

Will firefighters resist the option to manually take protected elevators out of service as they have appropriately done in the past, thereby overriding the emergency operations mode? Taking elevators out of service will slow an evacuation and increase the risk of entrapping occupants. Many firefighters are likely to distrust the technology, at least initially. Training will be required to increase trust.

Will occupants who are waiting for the elevator panic and endanger themselves by needlessly leaving elevator lobbies and using the stairs? Signage that estimates wait times until an elevator arrives could allay fear and panic. The technology is used for public transportation, and research indicates that wait times are more acceptable to riders when they are given such information. Elevator wardens can provide further reassurance.

Will developers and building owners assume the added expense of installing EOE elevator systems? The profitability of high-rise buildings is directly correlated to the amount of rentable or salable square footage. New code provisions have been enacted that would allow buildings over 420 feet in height to forgo the mandatory third stairs if the elevators were EOE enabled, providing a strong incentive for developers to install the systems.

5. **Fire-Service Access Elevators.** The process of climbing stairs is extremely arduous and time-consuming for firefighters and can interfere with and slow occupants descending stairs. They are burdened with heavy loads of personal protection equipment and must rest frequently. Emergency responders can override the normal operation of elevators, but normal elevators are vulnerable to the same hazards that endanger building occupants. Codes in the United States now require new buildings taller than 130 feet to have protected elevators dedicated to the use of emergency responders. Such dedicated fire-service access elevators have been a required feature in new high-rise buildings in Europe for the last few decades.

While similar to the requirements that protect emergency elevators for occupant evacuations, fire-service access elevators are restricted from occupant use and dedicated to the fire service. Unlike emergency occupant evacuation elevators, the routing of fire-service access elevators is not automated.

## New Approaches to Managing Emergency Responses in High-Rise Buildings

Research on the behavior of building occupants has clearly revealed that building occupants do not generally start evacuating a building soon after the fire alarm sounds. Rather, many occupants delay action pending a better understanding about whether the emergency is real or just a false alarm. It was once common to wait for responding firefighters to manage the evacuation by ordering people to move and by directing some occupants to evacuate while other occupants are expected to remain where they are already located. However, given how quickly a fire emergency can evolve, these delays have proven unacceptable.

Efforts are thus underway to initiate effective action prior to the arrival of the fire department. New York City has been at the vanguard of mandating improvement in the way that emergencies are managed in tall buildings. As early as 1973, New York City introduced Local Law 5, which mandated a certified Fire Safety Director (FSD) on duty in high-rise business buildings. These persons were responsible for the life safety of the occupants within the buildings and have expertise in utilizing fire-protection systems. The requirement was extended in 1980s to include high-rise hotels.

In response to 9/11, New York City again extended the requirements beyond fires to all types of hazards. Emergency Action Plan (EAP) directors are hired by building owners or managers and are charged with the duties of devising emergency action plans, training emergency response teams and building occupants, and directing occupant actions and evacuations during emergency operations.[11] Other cities have followed suit, including Chicago, Seattle, San Francisco, and Los Angeles.

In the continuing effort to professionalize responsibilities for emergency responses in tall building as well as other complex structures, the National Fire Protection Association (NFPA) published an all-hazard guide for emergency action plan development in high-rise office buildings.[12] Its efforts are ongoing, with an NFPA technical committee now charged with writing a model standard for qualifying Emergency Action Plan (EAP) directors for all types of structures.

Recent innovations in how to better manage occupants during emergencies has included a heuristic model designed to help operational managers decide which building occupants should be located where during an emergency.[13] It has also included a situation awareness information requirement analysis that anticipates the information needs of people who must make critical actionable decisions during an emergency.[14]

## Improving Safety in Tall Buildings Internationally

Tall buildings are being constructed throughout the world. The United States and Europe have been at the forefront of improving the safety of tall buildings, but not necessarily in the forefront of building very tall buildings. In particular, many very tall buildings have been constructed in both East Asia and the Middle East. Building codes in developing countries in these regions generally lag behind the more stringent standards adopted in the West, and enforcing building codes has proven questionable in some countries. The means for protecting these buildings are not generally publicized, but two problematic features are apparent.

Until recently, most tall buildings in the Middle East were constructed with flammable facades. To increase design flexibility and insulation as well as reduce costs, polyurethane was sandwiched between aluminum panels that were attached to the exterior of these buildings. Numerous high-rise fires in the Middle East and East Asia have been propagated along the exterior of buildings with this feature; for example, this occurred in several buildings in Dubai.[15] Because these fires spread along the exterior of buildings, there have been few fatalities to date, although the resulting monetary losses have been enormous.

One glaring exception has been the 2017 Grenfell Tower disaster in London, resulting in seventy-one fatalities. Like most disastrous fires, the fatalities cannot be attributed to a single fault. The lack of sprinklers and an alarm system, a single exit stairway, and the flammable exterior cladding all contributed to the disaster. Other fires have not yielded the same terrible results despite the rapidly burning exteriors because additional fire protection features were in place and because they often occurred in buildings with far fewer occupants. The costs of retrofitting building in Britain are thought to be enormous. An estimated eighty-two high-rise towers in Britain have similarly flammable exterior cladding.[16]

This type of fire has not been problematic in the United States, where codes prohibit such flammable exteriors.[17] Although such material has also been prohibited in the United Arab Emirates since 2013, an estimated 70 percent of the existing tall buildings in the United Arab Emirates have this feature.

China has adopted the practice of requiring a refuge floor in its tall buildings. In these buildings, an entire floor is a dedicated location where occupants can rest before continuing their evacuation. This approach, which is not used in the United States, is not without critics.[18] Refuge floors are open to the exterior of the building on two sides, which can provide fresh air to the refuge floor but can also potentially allow smoke from a fire on lower floors to make at least part of the refuge floor untenable. Moreover, the approach greatly reduces the rentable square footage in the building, and it may be that it is more cost-effective to spend funds in enhancing other fire protective building features. Inspections of refuge floors have revealed problems in dedicating the required floor space to occupants and in providing for the relative comfort of occupants during longer-term stays, since seating and sanitary facilities are not required.

## Conclusion: Are Tall Buildings Safe?

This chapter has cataloged numerous improvements in the safety of occupants in high-rise buildings. It is clear that—at least in the United States and Europe—we are safer than ever in routine fire emergencies. These improvements also increase the likelihood that occupants are more likely to survive terrorist attacks.

While beyond the scope of this chapter, security improvement in signature high-rise buildings has also been greatly enhanced, decreasing the likelihood that attackers can sneak into buildings with explosives. However, risk has not been eliminated. Terrorists can innovate new ways to attack and the costs of protecting tall buildings from all possible scenarios is prohibitive. And economic pressures to reduce the costs of constructing high-rise buildings remain, with the potential for disastrous results. The Grenfell Tower disaster resulted from the failure to adequately regulate fire protection features and cost scores of lives in Britain.[19] Still, it seems that we are indeed safer occupying tall buildings than in the past.

## Notes

1. Bob Lewis, "East Coast Earthquake Strongest Since 1944," Associated Press, August 23, 2011.

2. John Handley, "*Terrorist Attack Fear Not Tallest Spire's Toughest Test,*" *Chicago Tribune,* July 27, 2005.

3. Acitelli, 2006; Brenzel, 2016; World Economic News, "Terrorism vs. Tourism," November 20, 2001; Jad Mouawad, "Dip in Tourism After Most Attacks Is Short-Lived," *New York Times,* November 30, 2015; CNN, "*New York Sees Record Number of Tourists in 2012,*" January 1, 2013. https://goo.gl/1TU5HP; Michael Saul Howard, "New York City Sees Record High Tourism in 2013," *Wall Street Journal,* December 10, 2013.

4. Hall, 2013.

5. NIST, 2011.

6. International Code Council, 2011.

7. Averill, 2005.

8. Ibid., 152.

9. American Society of Mechanical Engineers, 1991, 1995.

10. Groner, 2002.

11. Fire Safety Directors Association of Greater New York, 2016.

12. High-Rise Building Safety Advisory Committee, 2014.

13. Groner, 2015.

14. Groner, 2009.

15. Ramona Ruiz, "Experts Query Quality of Cladding on Dubai Buildings," *The National* (Dubai), January 1, 2016.

16. Reuters World Service, "UK Announces Fire Safety Review after Tests Identify 82 Unsafe Tower Blocks," July 28, 2017.

17. Bill Law, "'Towering Inferno' Fears for Gulf's High-Rise Blocks," BBC News, May 2, 2013; Valiulis, 2015.

18. O'Conner, Clawson, and Cui, 2012.

19. David D. Kirkpatrick, Danny Hakim, and James Glanz, "Why Grenfell Tower Burned: Regulators Put Cost before Safety," *New York Times,* June 24, 2017.

## References

Acitelli, Tom. "The New Building Boom." December 1 2006. https://goo.gl/az4swx.

American Society of Mechanical Engineers. *Elevators, Fire Accessibility Proceedings.* New York: American Society of Mechanical Engineers, 1995.

———. *Symposium on Elevators and Fire Proceedings.* New York: American Society of Mechanical Engineers, 1991.

Averill, Jason D., et al. *Occupant Behavior, Egress, and Emergency Communications: Federal Building and Fire Safety Investigation of the World Trade Center Disaster.* Gaithersburg, MD: National Institute of Standards and Technology, 2005.

Brenzel, Kathryn. *The Future of NYC Real Estate.* New York: New York Real Estate News, 2016.

Fire Safety Directors Association of Greater New York. *FSD/EAP Director Overview.* New York: Fire Safety Directors Association of Greater New York, 2016.

Groner, Norman. "A Compelling Case for Emergency Elevator Systems." *Fire Engineering* 155, no. 10 (2002): 126–128.

———. "A Situation Awareness Requirements Analysis for the Use of Elevators During Fire Emergencies." *International Symposium on Human Behaviour in Fire,* 61–72. Cambridge: Interscience Communications, 2009.

———. "A Simple Decision Model for Managing the Movement of Building Occupants during Fire Emergencies." *5th International Symposium on Human Behaviour in Fire: Conference Proceedings,* 47–55. London: Interscience Communications, 2015.

Hall, John. *High-Rise Building Fire.* Quincy, MA: National Fire Protection Association, 2013.

High-Rise Building Safety Advisory Committee. *Guidelines to Developing Emergency Action Plans for All-Hazard Emergencies in High-Rise Office Buildings.* Quincy, MA: National Fire Protection Association, 2014.

International Code Council. *Building Safety Codes Changed as a Result of 9/11.* Washington, DC: International Code Council, 2011.

NIST. *World Trade Center Disaster Study Recommendations.* New York: NIST, 2011.

O'Conner, D., K. Clawson, and E. Cui. "Considerations and Challenges in Refuge Areas in Tall Buildings." *CTBUH 9th International Conference.* Shanghai: CTBUH, 2012.

The Skyscraper Center. https://goo.gl/KJmkCQ.

Valiulis, John. "Building Exterior Wall Assembly Flammability: Have We Forgotten the Past 40 Years?" *Fire Engineering*, November 24, 2015.

# Health Impacts of 9/11

Michael Crane, Kimberly Flynn, Roberto Lucchini,
Guille Mejia, Jacqueline Moline, David Prezant,
Joan Reibman, and Micki Siegel de Hernández,
with Cristina Onea and Susan Opotow*

The attacks on World Trade Center's Twin Towers by nineteen terrorists on September 11, 2001, caused severe damage, fires, and the
collapse of those two iconic buildings in Lower Manhattan. Almost three
thousand people were killed, and more than six thousand others were
wounded that day. The buildings' collapse produced tons of toxic rubble
and a dense dust cloud that exposed thousands of people to toxins.[1] Over
time, workers on the site, including first responders, recovery, and cleanup
workers; people who lived, worked, and attended school in the vicinity;
and visitors to the site on 9/11 developed chronic and sometimes fatal
illnesses that included declines in pulmonary function and an elevated
risk of heart disease, as well as various kinds of cancer.[2] This also resulted
in an elevated risk of posttraumatic stress disorder, behavioral problems
for exposed youth,[3] and other mental health illnesses from being caught
up in, witnessing the attacks or its horrifying sequelae, or experiencing
personal loss in its aftermath.

In April 2016, eight people—doctors, labor unionists, and community
activists—met to describe the significant health-related issues and the
medical, logistical, political, and policy issues that arose after 9/11. They
recounted the public health challenges that emerged and how civic agencies at the city, state, and federal level responded to them over time. They
also described the formation of initiatives and coalitions among various
experts in occupational health, unions representing first responders, response and recovery workers, and workers in the affected areas, people
living and working near the World Trade Center, and elected officials.

**145**

Although the efforts of these groups were initially rebuffed, various civic entities became allies.

Ultimately, after continuous advocacy for almost a decade, Congress passed the James Zadroga 9/11 Health and Compensation Act in 2010. The legislation was reauthorized in 2015 and signed by President Barack Obama. The "Zadroga Act," as it is commonly called, provides medical monitoring and treatment for certain 9/11-related health conditions for responders, survivors, and volunteers affected by the September 11 attacks, as well as financial compensation for eligible individuals for some physical health conditions or death due to 9/11 illnesses. The Zadroga Act also established the federally funded World Trade Center Health Program (WTCHP). Administered by the National Institute for Occupational Safety and Health (NIOSH), the September 11th Victim Compensation Fund (VCF), and the Department of Justice (DOJ), it is attentive to the well-being of individuals and communities affected by the 2001 attacks in New York City; Shanksville, Pennsylvania; the Pentagon; and the country as a whole.

Attentive to multiple levels—individuals, communities, the city, the state, and the nation—this chapter's analyses of 9/11's aftermath over an extended period, based on medical knowledge and direct experience, offers insight into: the various kinds of health-related trauma experienced after a devastating attack;[4] the responses of governmental entities at the local, state, and national levels; the mobilization of individuals and groups in response to the health challenges and fears they faced; and the relevance of this tragic event for preparedness in the future.[5] It offers aggregated and experientially based information about acute and chronic individual and public health issues, and concludes with a discussion of what can be learned from the 9/11 postdisaster trajectory and with an epilogue on emerging issues.

## Contamination and Negation: Emerging Health Problems after 9/11

**Jacqueline Moline**: Early on there were tremendous obstacles to addressing post–9/11 health problems. The biggest obstacle, in many ways, was the City of New York City itself. It was a huge challenge when Dr. Thomas Frieden, the New York City Health Commissioner at that time,[6] was not convinced that there were any health sequelae from the World Trade Center attacks nor that reported health conditions were real or would persist. Ironically, the most authoritative data on post–9/11 health conditions were being aggregated by another New York City agency—the Fire Department of New York (FDNY). Yet, in spite of the FDNY's alarming data, it was tremendously challenging to get an acknowledgement of the severity of an emerging health crisis. It took several years and lots of data collection to get the City to finally accept that there were significant emerging health problems that needed to be addressed. What caused this change? Partly the data, partly persistence, and partly three groups that came together: (1) a city agency, the Fire Department of New York; (2) the tremendous community of residents from downtown; and (3) the union and medical responder communities. Together, they argued: "We're all saying the same thing. You can't discount this. It isn't—as you've claimed—'just PTSD.'" The groups' coming together enabled a shift so that programs began to emerge to address post–9/11 problems in New York City.

**David Prezant**: I spent many days in the US Congress fighting for money from the federal government for these medical programs and educating various congressional staffers. We did this year after year. We were asked the same questions again and again: "Why [this or that agency] isn't paying for that?" "Where is the data?" And local challenges were just as difficult. It felt like you were fighting from within at the same time you were lobbying Congress for money. You had local government that took a narrow, parochial standpoint and asked, "Who's going to be responsible for the cleanup?" "Is it the city's responsibility or is it a federal responsibility?" This resulted in much infighting. Ultimately, the denial that there was a problem at both city and federal levels intensified post–9/11 health problems.

**Micki Siegel de Hernández** (Labor unionist): The ongoing problem with accountability was a major barrier and constituted a failed public health response to a significant public health problem that impacted responders, area workers, residents, schoolchildren, and other community members. Saying this was a "failed" public health response is not even accurate because it suggests that measures were taken to protect the public that were not effective. There were no such measures. Many health and environmental experts knew what the primary components of the contamination and fires were, or what was possibly there, and the potential health effects that could result from exposures, but this knowledge was, unfortunately, negated, ignored, and lied about by government agencies. So the advocacy that we all were involved with was not just about getting money for the health program. We wanted the health conditions recognized as related to 9/11 exposures, and we wanted the extent of the contamination recognized and addressed.

To bring attention to these issues required persistence—holding agencies' feet to the fire—to get these problems recognized. Remember, this was during President George Bush's administration (1/20/2001–1/20/2009) and then Mayor Rudolph Giuliani in New York City. Initially and over the years that followed 9/11, there were many examples of health information and health "alerts" put out by the government that minimized or ignored the toxic nature of the contaminants, the extent of the contamination, the potential, negative health effects of exposures, and the communities at risk. In the midst of this tragedy and public health disaster, you had the head of the EPA assuring everyone that the air in New York City was safe to breathe and Mayor Giuliani opening up the downtown area six days after the attacks and urging New Yorkers to come downtown to "go shopping." That message from the government—that everything was "fine" in terms of exposures and there was nothing to worry about—persisted, even when health issues began to emerge and be reported. On the local level, the information provided to the public by the New York City Department of Health was pathetic and minimized the potential for exposures and health impacts, even for pregnant women. Although we were eventually able to secure funding for the WTC Health Program and the VCF, we were never successful in getting the issues related to contamination and exposures addressed satisfactorily. There was never an adequate assessment by the government of 9/11 contamination in the impacted areas. There wasn't even appropriate guidance provided. Building owners, landlords, business owners, employers, and the public were essentially on their own.

**Guille Mejia**: It was a huge challenge to get the city to recognize that there was going to be a problem that resulted from environmental conditions at Ground Zero[7] that responders and volunteers faced. The New York City Office of Labor Relations refused to classify Ground Zero as a hazardous waste site. As a result, many extant worker protection laws and regulations did not apply and could not be enforced. That led to major and continued exposures. So we had to deal with such questions as: How do you classify this incident and how do you define it? How do you control some of the things that are happening there? Meanwhile, we had to deal with Mayor Rudy Giuliani, who wanted to open up the city a week after 9/11 and said, "Everything is fine."

**Prezant:** He did open it up. Six days later.

**Mejia:** Right, and as a result of that decision, more and more people were exposed unnecessarily. There was much conflicting information and many groups involved, which hindered timely responses to the emerging questions and concerns from workers. For example, DC 37 is a public-sector labor organization with 121,000 members. There were numerous tasks required to advance the many phases of rescue, recovery, and cleanup work at Ground Zero and the surrounding area in Lower Manhattan. The number of city employees needed went beyond the uniformed services. For example, New York City Department of Transportation and New York Police Department motor vehicle operators carted off debris as workers desperately worked to dig out and recover bodies. Traffic enforcement agents were needed to secure access to the site and surrounding streets. Engineers had to determine the structural integrities of the buildings in and around Ground Zero. Morgue technicians were needed to remove bodies and assist in their identification. City chaplains comforted distraught workers as they dealt with the death and destruction surrounding them. Public health nurses provided medical assistance to those injured on 9/11 and in the months that followed.

Since the WTC complex is situated in the financial center of New York City and in the heart of city governance, public sector workers—many of whom were DC 37 members—were dispatched to their office buildings to recover necessary business and equipment to keep the city government running. Some of our members returned to their offices within days of the building collapse only to find out the buildings had not been properly decontaminated.

**Moline:** In 1993, after the first bombing of the World Trade Center, the Port Authority of New York and New Jersey called the Department of Preventive Medicine at Mount Sinai Hospital to ask us if we could provide 24/7 coverage at the World Trade Center. They particularly wanted us to provide respiratory clearance examinations for all federal and state personnel who would be evaluating the bomb crater because they knew there was asbestos. In 1993 we arranged twenty-four-hour coverage and provided basic exams to be sure workers' blood pressure was within normal limits so that they could safely wear a respirator to go on site.

Having assisted in this way in 1993, we called the Port Authority on September 12, 2001, to offer similar services. I had the entire Mount Sinai Hospital Department of Medicine ready to go with people lined up for 24/7 coverage. Everyone had volunteered to do this. But the New York City Department of Health said: "No. We don't want people to come down"—because they were concerned about liability. We had done this eight years before, and the Port Authority had no issue. They had called us! Then, when we offered to do the exact same thing, when we said, "Let's do what we did before," not knowing the scale that it was going to be—they said, "No. We don't want to do it because we don't know what we would tell people if we found some symptoms." They just put a kibosh on it. We weren't allowed to go down and even do a basic respirator clearance exam.[8] That's the kind of pushback we got early on from the New York City Department of Health. This was obstruction. If you weren't right in there you wouldn't believe how challenging it was to be fighting for everything tooth and nail.

## "Clean It Up Yourself"

In the wake of the September 11 attacks and the implosion of the World Trade Center Towers, adults and children living, working, and attending school in Lower Manhattan faced urgent questions concerning health—both short- and long-term—in their homes, workplaces, and schools, as well as mental health issues. But the answers they received from governmental entities at the local level from the New York City Department of Health and at the federal level from the US Environmental Protection Agency were evasive or misstated the available information. Eventually this led to legal challenges in order to demand that these agencies attend to the health of the public rather than political and economic interests.

**Kimberly Flynn**: I'm going to briefly take us back in time to an important obstructive moment, something mentioned by Micki, because it is a critical piece of the lessons learned. Not long after 9/11, the New York City Department of Health issued a public health advisory concerning air quality near the World Trade Center site, in the form of Frequently Asked Questions. It was referenced among survivors as the "Clean It Up Yourself FAQs" or the "Fah-Qs to Downtown Residents." It instructs you to clean your apartment yourself with a wet rag and run your air conditioner on recirculate. Here's the final FAQ. The question: "Do pregnant women and young children need to take additional precautions?" The answer: "No. Pregnant women and young children do not need to take additional precautions."

This is evidence of willful denial. It's beyond implausible to claim that the developing fetus would not be susceptible to harm from exposure to this level of pollution. The EPA had to know that. There were people at the City Health Department who knew that. And by 2004, we had scientific evidence that this advice was false and reckless.[9]

We also know that residents and workers have PTSD from coming under attack by Al Qaeda; of course, many did and still do. But having been to many, many community meetings after 9/11, I will tell you that people were made three times crazier than they needed to be by essentially being told: "There's no problem here. Suck it up. People died in those buildings. Why are you complaining about a cough? Go get a wet rag and clean it up yourself." And people who did that started to have health problems, like those who returned to Battery Park City and started to clean up their residences. When they complained of symptoms like breathing problems or scratched corneas from getting WTC dust in their eyes, they were basically told, "These problems have nothing to do with 9/11."

**Joan Reibman**: In other words, the message was, "Everyone gets asthma anyway."

**Flynn:** New York City has a high baseline asthma rate, and that was thrown back at us by the New York City Department of Health (DOH). Then, when it became clear that a lot of people were having new or worsened respiratory problems, the DOH said these were strictly the result of temporary irritation and would disappear as soon as the fires on the pile were out. Because the affected residents are New Yorkers, they're not shy, and they figure that they can get the DOH on the phone. And when they called, they literally were sent in a circle from the DOH to the City Department of Environment Protection, which then sent them on to the New York State Department of Environmental Conservation, which sent them to the Environmental Protection Agency (EPA) Region 2, which sent them back to the

# Public Health Advisory Concerning Air Quality in the Affected Area of the World Trade Center Disaster

The NYC Department of Health (DOH), in collaboration with the City, State, and Federal agencies, is closely monitoring and analyzing air quality data in the wake of the World Trade Center disaster. Following the collapse of the Twin Towers, significant quantities of smoke and dust have been released into the air. The plume of smoke contained dust, ash, soot, and other burning materials present at the site.

In general, dusts can cause respiratory symptoms and eye and throat irritation. Because dust will continue to remain in the air during the ensuing clean-up efforts following the World Trade Center disaster, residents in the vicinity of the World Trade Center are encouraged to take precautions when they return to their homes.

### What are the Recommendations for Residents Living in Lower Manhattan?
All residents in the immediate vicinity of the World Trade Center - particularly those who live the area bounded by Warren Street to the North, Broadway to the East, the Hudson River to the West, and Exchange and Thames Streets to the South - should take the following precautions when they return to their homes:

- Avoid unnecessary outdoor strenuous activity;
- Avoid sweeping or other outdoor maintenance;
- Keep dust from entering the home (e.g., remove shoes before entering the home);
- Keep windows closed;
- Set the air conditioner to recirculate air (closed vents), and clean or change the filter frequently;

### What should I do if I experience respiratory symptoms?
Dust and other particulate matter have the greatest impact on persons with underlying respiratory conditions. Such individuals may experience chest tightness, wheezing, and shortness of breath. Anyone who has difficulty breathing should consult their physicians, especially those with underlying respiratory conditions. People with asthma may need to increase their usual medical treatment with more frequent use of bronchodilators, and should consult their physicians if necessary.

### If I experience any eye irritation what should I do?
Ocular saline solutions or tap water may be used to rinse eyes irritated by dust. All persons should avoid wearing contact lenses while in the affected area.

### What are the health effects of asbestos?
Destruction of the World Trade Center buildings released large amounts of dust and ash, some of which contained trace amounts of asbestos. Based on the asbestos test results received thus far, the general public's risk for any short or long term adverse health affects are extremely low.

In general, asbestos-related lung disease general results only from intense asbestos exposure experienced over a period of many years, primarily as a consequence of occupational exposures. The risk of developing an asbestos-related illness following an exposure of short duration is very low.

### What measures are being taken to protect the rescue workers?
Rescue workers have been equipped with half-face masks, goggles, and protective clothing to reduce their exposure to dust and other particulate matter while working in the blast zone.

### How can I clean up dusts in or near my home or office?
The best way to remove dust is to use a wet rag or wet mop. Sweeping with a dry broom is not recommended because it can make dust airborne again. Dirty rags should be put in plastic bags while they are still wet and bags should be sealed and discarded (cloth rags can be washed, see instructions below). Rags should not be allowed to dry out before bagging and disposal or washing. Because the dust particles are so small, standard vacuuming is not an efficient way to remove the dust. High efficiency vacuums, which are now widely available in stores, should be used to remove dust. Carpets and upholstery can be shampooed, then vacuumed.

Persons should shower to rinse off any dust from hair and skin. Dusty clothes should be washed separately from other clothing. Pets can be washed with running water from a hose or faucet; their paws should be wiped to avoid tracking dust inside the home. To clean plants, rinse leaves with water. Throw away any food that may have been contaminated with dust. Food in cans, jars or containers with tight-fitting lids do not need to be discarded. However, if there is dust present on the exterior of vacuum-sealed food containers, just wash the can or jar with water and wipe it clean. **If in doubt, throw it out.**

Air purifiers may help reduce indoor dust levels. High efficiency air purifiers are superior to other models in filtering the smallest particles. Air purifiers are only useful for removing dust from the air. They will not remove dust already deposited on floors, shelves, upholstery or rugs. Keep windows closed when using an air purifier.

### Do pregnant women and young children need to take additional precautions?
No. Pregnant women and young children do not need to take additional precautions.

*Go to* WTC Information page || NYC DOH Home Page || Health Topics || Public Information ||
NYC.gov Home Page || Mayor's Office || City Agencies || Services || News and Features || City Life || Contact Us || Search

Figure 1. Public Health Advisory concerning air quality.

DOH. Everywhere people turned, there were no answers they could trust. There was denial, and there was also an endless runaround. And people became completely incensed by this.

At one point, I was in a meeting in Battery Park City, and I started talking to them about asbestos because that was the only thing the government would cop to at that point. We knew there were regulations around asbestos, so we went with asbestos. We were later criticized by Laurie Garrett, a science journalist, for doing that.[10] But at that point, we were answering the government's admission that there was asbestos, just not enough of it to be a problem. So we were disputing the claim that asbestos was present at "safe" levels.

When I was talking to residents about asbestos, there was an ethnographer sitting in the back of the room taking notes. And at a certain point, one of the residents—with whom I later became good friends—became enraged with me and said, "You environmentalists! What are you doing here?" He said, "We don't need you. I'm going to pick up the phone and I'm going to call Sheldon Silver,[11] and he's going to help us, so we don't need you here talking to us about risks at all."

At the meeting's end, the ethnographer came up to me and said, "Does this happen often?" I said, "It happened because I'm giving them some very bad news. Not only am I saying, 'Look there could be a problem with the stuff that's in your living rooms and your workplaces and the carpet your kid crawls on,' but I'm also saying to them, 'Sheldon Silver's probably not going to be able to get you out of this one.'" And one of the things that happened in that meeting—and I started to repeat at other meetings—is that I said to them: "Call Sheldon Silver. Call everyone you think might be able to help. But at the end of the day, if you don't get what you need, here's my cell phone number. Call me. Because it might come down to us." And it did come down to us—the people on the ground—to fight for a proper cleanup. I would never have thought that it would have taken such an enormous effort, with years of organizing, cultivating relationships with independent experts, gathering evidence, and building pressure. And thank goodness we did build a coalition because we needed it. We worked with community groups across Lower Manhattan from river to river—the Hudson River to the East River—and we worked with the New York Committee for Occupational Safety and Health (NYCOSH) and the unions.

Community advocates working with NYCOSH[12] opened the way for the formation of an incredible network with labor unions. And it was this coalition—the World Trade Center Community Labor Coalition—that took on the US Environmental Protection Agency (EPA) during the public meetings of the EPA Expert Technical Review Panel, which met in Lower Manhattan in 2004–2005 to address unmet 9/11 health needs. Those unmet needs included assessing and addressing what WTC contamination remained in downtown homes, schools, and workplaces. We never got what we fought for in the panel process: the new, scientifically valid EPA Test and Clean Program. And we were outraged that the EPA squandered yet another opportunity to protect human health by preventing chronic exposures to WTC indoor contamination. However, we did emerge with strengthened intergroup relationships that took us into the next phase—the push for federally funded WTC health care for the downtown community as well as for responders.

Overall, the way the government mishandled the 9/11 environmental aftermath was retraumatizing for the community. People had come under attack from terrorists and needed to believe in their government. They needed to believe that their government could and would protect them. Many absolutely could not take in the message that the government lied to them about what they were being exposed to and was denying them the help that they needed to be safe. This feeling of betrayal persists and shows no sign of abating.

**Prezant:** Residents and landlords owned apartments in Lower Manhattan. Some could have moved but didn't want to for a variety of reasons.

**Flynn:** You have to understand that people were told it was safe. They were told early and they were told often: "It's safe. It's not a problem." The majority of Battery Park City residents were rent-paying tenants, and many desperately tried to break their leases and ended up being sued in Housing Court by their landlords; or they sued their landlords to force them to do a proper cleanup. In either case, the whole thing was a debacle and tenants were the losers.

These days, the west side of Lower Manhattan has many multimillion-dollar condos, but that was not the case fifteen years ago. There were people in rent-stabilized or public housing who simply could not afford to move. A similar dynamic played out at Stuyvesant High School, located a few blocks north of Ground Zero. The Parents Association divided down the middle on whether the school was safe for students to reoccupy. The parents who were convinced that the school was safe told the parents who weren't convinced that they should find another school. Pulling your child out of Stuyvesant was depriving them of an education at one of the country's highest ranked high schools. Though many parents were worried about residual contamination in the school, only one family chose to leave Stuyvesant that I know of. Later testing conducted by an environmental consultant hired by the school's parent association revealed that parents' concerns were warranted. In particular, the auditorium, which had been heavily used by responders during the early days of the cleanup, was loaded with asbestos and lead.

**Reibman:** Of course people wanted to come back to their home. It's their home. And of course people wanted to go back to their work. It's their livelihood. So you can't blame people for that. At those community meetings early on, a mother stood up and said: "Just tell me, is it safe for me to take my child back?" When they were told, "Yes," or "We don't really know but you might as well go back," first of all, they went crazy. And if you want to talk long term, to this day, one of the issues we have is that parents who went back—who brought their kids back because it was their home—may have wanted go somewhere else but did not have the money and were told it was okay to go back. Now they say, "Did I put my kid at risk? "And do I now have to worry for the next $x$ number of years that my kid is going to be at risk for, at the least, sinus disease, but at the worst, cancer?" So there's a deep-rooted concern and guilt that goes with what you saw in those parents then and you still see now.

## Mental Health Issues as Uncompensated Injury

**Michael Crane**: Let's talk about ongoing issues with mental health and 9/11. People with mental health conditions have been discriminated against in spite of the certainty that 9/11 was a devastating experience. Maybe it was all the death, maybe it was all the grief, but even among governmental experts, there was a differentiation between people with medical conditions and people with mental health conditions. The proof of this is that that the September 11th Victim Compensation Fund provided no compensation for 9/11-caused mental health issues. They were not funded to pay for it. It was not part of the deal. If you have lung disease, you can get reimbursed for illness. But mental health conditions got left out, and this was among the most prevalent conditions and the most damaging.

**Siegel de Hernández**: There was tremendous pushback in Congress, mostly by Republicans, for 9/11 funding. Those opposed to the Victim Compensation Fund (VCF) objected to funding compensation for mental health conditions from the very beginning. Opponents said, "Well, everybody could have mental health problems." So mental health was not covered in the VCF. It was wrong, but it was part of the political process that included opposition to funding.

**Crane:** It was easier to talk about the injuries that seemed to have emerged or worsened by the World Trade Center exposure, but there were other problems. There are preexisting, postexisting conditions, and there is now greater sensitivity to transgenerational problems. A father became ill and something happened to the child as a result. I am not a psychiatrist, but this separation of fundable and unfundable injury is one of those things that just stun me about the 9/11 program and about the United States.

## Challenging the U.S. Environmental Protection Agency

**Flynn:** In 2008, Lower Manhattan residents, students, and workers eventually did file suit against the US Environmental Protection Agency (EPA) in the US District Court for the Southern District of New York, making a claim based on the Fifth Amendment to the Constitution that prohibits the government from leading citizens into harm's way. The EPA then filed a motion for summary judgment to get the suit dismissed. Presiding Judge Deborah Batts issued an astonishing decision that said that the EPA's claim that the air was safe to breathe "shocked the conscience,"[13] and she denied the EPA motion for dismissal, saying, "No, no. The case should go forward."

A number of us were present at the final court hearing on the case and heard the attorney for the EPA get up and make arguments that the federal government has a legitimate interest in preserving its right to mislead citizens during and after a disaster if there are "competing concerns" like reopening the New York Stock Exchange. We walked out of that hearing saying, "Oh my God." What we had heard meant to us that the government reserves the right to lie to the public in the aftermath of an environmental disaster. We later learned that two of the three appellate judges agreed with that argument. That was our takeaway.

**Siegel de Hernández**: Some sampling data were collected by agencies such as the US Environmental Protection Agency (EPA), which had published evidence contrary to what they subsequently claimed. The early environmental sampling data from the EPA mysteriously disappeared from their website. And that is partly how we pushed those agencies—by using their own information. We'd say: "This is what you wrote in this document. Why are you now saying that that's not a problem?" There were many people who were sick because of their exposures. Much of this could have been prevented, particularly once rescue operations became response and recovery operations. So much more could have been done then that would have mitigated the extent of those health impacts now.

**Moline:** The most shocking and revealing thing to look at what the EPA actually wanted to say and what they were allowed to say as the result of memos that were edited by the White House. President George Bush's Council on Environmental Quality had a mindset along the lines of "chemicals are good for you" and "breathe all this bad stuff and you'll be fine," which was actually included in the edited version of the EPA document. You can see what the EPA wanted to say and the White House revisions.[14] When the revisions to the EPA report were made public in a scathing report by US EPA Inspector General Nikki Tinsley, she was fired. This was how the process worked. An agency may speak the truth but not when competing interests are considered. Key financial markets were collocated near the disaster, and the well-being of those markets prevailed over the health of people who lived and worked there. And this will happen again if need be. That's just the reality in the aftermath of disaster. It gives you a reality check.

All of us are striving to do what we think is right for the public. Yet, we're being told, "You may be doing what's right but you can't do it because that isn't as important to us as the business we're in." I had an opportunity to read the transcript of someone who works for the New York City Buildings Department. He was asked some questions about 9/11 and, under oath, he claimed that there were no health problems related to 9/11—despite being confronted with hundreds of studies. And this deposition occurred in 2016, fifteen years after the 9/11 attacks! Interests that competed with public health remained influential throughout the years after 2001.

## Lessons Learned in the Aftermath of 9/11

Looking back over the past decade and a half, the experts discussed lessons learned about protecting public health in the aftermath of the September 11 attacks.[15] This section reports on five of these lessons. Though these examples are from New York City, these principles have wider relevance.

### 1. The Importance of Data: Health Registries

**Prezant:** Some of those we saw as adversaries early on ultimately became critical partners, and we wouldn't have accomplished what we did without data from the New York City Department of Health. Survivors would not have had a strong argument. Joan [Reibman; Medical Director, World Trade Center Environmental Health Center] did not have enough data. She was treating people from the community, but she wasn't looking at 100,000 people. New York City Department of Health World Trade Center Health Registry ("Registry") became our critical partners. We wouldn't have accomplished what we did without them.

**Siegel de Hernández:** I agree that in the early years after 9/11, there were constant struggles with the City of New York. With the clarity of hindsight, some groups like the Registry did indeed become critical. But in the early years after 9/11, there was a lot of fighting with the City of New York. It was an endless push to get them to the point where they recognized the link between 9/11–related exposures and the existence of post–9/11 health conditions. The city government finally got to a place where it could no longer deny the mountain of evidence that was being amassed. So such initiatives as the Registry have a long and conflicted history. It is important to remember that every, positive step forward was the result of a protracted battle.

The proposal to fund the Registry, which would be run by the NYC Department of Health and Mental Hygiene, came several years after 9/11. The hypothesis included in the proposal for funding the Registry was that there would be no long-term health effects of 9/11. Because of that and because of the way that the city had downplayed the potential for exposures and denied the existence of 9/11-related illnesses up to that point, the Registry lacked widespread support when it began. This significantly impacted the number of people who enrolled in the Registry. The Registry could have been a much better resource with a larger pool of enrollees if the agencies involved had worked collaboratively with the community and labor organizations from its inception. It could have had more support and many more participants, particularly from labor organizations that did not trust NYC's intent. Many labor unions, coordinated by the New York State AFL-CIO,[16] met with the head of the funding agency, the Agency for Toxic Substances and Disease Registry, and New York City representatives to raise specific concerns about the Registry's design and to request that changes be made before the first survey was distributed. Those requests were ignored. The Registry data did indeed become a very important source of information over time, but its scope remained limited because of problems early on.

## 2. The Importance of Raising Unwelcome Questions

**Siegel de Hernández**: At the beginning, because 9/11 was the horrible disaster that it was, everybody was in different mindset. Thousands of people had been killed, there was an ongoing rescue, and there was significant trauma. One of the challenges at that time, especially for those of us involved in advocacy, was that any kind of advocacy was viewed as un-American. There was a very different mindset at that stressful time about which issues could and could not be raised. This made advocacy especially difficult. And, at the same time, we were all suffering from those same issues, having lost people in our unions or families.

But we recognized that there was a separate, important problem that needed to be addressed. I don't think it is unusual after environmental disasters for agencies to be unwilling to address emerging health issues or to minimize what those issues are. Look at any environmental disaster and you see groups rising up because of health concerns that are not being addressed. Look at the destruction and deaths caused by Hurricane Katrina in New Orleans, Louisiana, in 2005. Many groups arose to protest the environmental impacts. That's just one example of many.

If there was another disaster tomorrow in New York City that had some environmental component, such as a dirty bomb,[17] I am not convinced that things would be any different. Maybe here in New York City we will be a little further along because of what we lived through and maybe we would have a head start on coalition building to start things off, but I think that we would still be raising unwelcome questions and fighting those battles about exposures and health risks. I don't think that we, as a country, have learned that lesson.

## 3. The Importance of Collaboration

**Reibman:** One of the things that you're seeing at this meeting is a coalition of disparate groups who took time to work together against external conflicts. We didn't always work together quite so beautifully as we do now because when there are not many crumbs, people fight hard for their own group. Look at the three groups that worked together. First, there was the Fire Department of New York (FDNY), the easiest group for people to support because, first of all, they had data. There was talk about needing data, but you don't have any data in a disaster. FDNY was the best place to get those data because they already had data collection protocols. So if any group was going to get support, it was the Fire Department of New York. Second, labor was already an organized group because of their unions. They had a battle to fight, and they already had organized processes programs for doing exactly that. Third was the community. The community has always been the stepchild because they had no preexisting organization. Ultimately they organized Beyond Ground Zero, a coalition of nine disparate groups based in Chinatown and the Lower East Side, and also 9/11 Environmental Action, which was largely residents and school parents on the west side of Lower Manhattan.[18]

Without a formal, overarching program, it took time for everyone to understand that by supporting each other, we were more likely have a better program for everyone. That is what we are describing now. It sounds great now—like we were a great coalition—but it took a long time to develop that. Forming a coalition is important. As you find yourself working against those who oppose your efforts, the first response is to be separate and compete for resources when in fact you need to work together.

# 9/11 ENVIRONMENTAL ACTION

*We are some of the many victims of the World Trade Center attack. On September 11th, 2002 an unprecedented amount of toxic materials rained down on the neighborhoods where we live, work and go to school. Asbestos, mercury, lead, VOCs and new combinations creating even more toxic substances blanketed the streets and buildings in the City we all love. As victims of a terrorist attack we also had to bear the burden of environmental testing and decontamination by ourselves. 9/11 ENVIRONMENTAL ACTION is our coalition of residents including representatives of the Lower Manhattan Tenants Coalition whose members number 15,000; worker safety experts; environmentalists; school parents and others concerned about our health. We believe that while the announcement that the EPA will clean downtown apartments represents a welcome change of heart, it does not go far enough.*

**In order for the cleanup to make Lower Manhattan safe again for our children, residents and workers our major challenge is to address these serious flaws in the EPA plan:**

- **EPA must agree to clean the inside of schools, workplaces, and commercial establishments.** Now the EPA will only agree to clean apartments. Children are the most vulnerable to illness from environmental toxins; they must be the most protected. EPA must be the lead agency responsible for the cleanup; all funding for the cleanup must go through the EPA.

- **The cleanup must go everywhere the giant plume of WTC smoke went**—that includes areas north of Canal Street, and even parts of Brooklyn and New Jersey. It also includes areas that were recontaminated by dust in the course of the cleanup of Ground Zero. Sufficient testing must be done to insure that all affected areas are included in the cleanup.

- **All indoor and outdoor areas must be remediated of all hazardous substances**, not just asbestos and fiberglass. Removal must be to the proper protocols with state-of-the-art technology.

- **Using visible dust as the indicator of contamination is unacceptable and scientifically invalid.** Fine and ultra-fine particulates cause long-term health risks that will create a new class of WTC victims for years and generations to come.

- **A medical registry and health surveillance system must be established for workers, residents, and students.**

- **All worker safety laws must be enforced in the cleanup operations.** People who work, live and visit our neighborhoods all have the same needs to be safe.

- **Mandatory cleanup should happen building by building not apartment to apartment**, so that dust does not cross -contaminate corridors and ductwork making our spaces unsafe once again.

- **Cleanup must operate in accordance with the principles of Environmental Justice**—omitting no income and/or ethnic group.

- **The office of the EPA National Ombudsman must be restored to its original independance.**

- **The National Contingency Plan must be enacted.** The NCP has the mechanisms and funding to make our demands happen.

**Please help us protect the health of the victims of this attack on America.**
To Contact the 9/11 Action Coalition call:

Figure 2. 9/11 Environmental Action, May 2002.

**Prezant:** Our work with the National Institute for Occupational Safety and Health (NIOSH) was a huge, behind-the-scenes success because NIOSH is an unusual agency that is very open to a collaborative relationship. They deal with stakeholders and because they've never been funded appropriately, they have developed an internal culture of working with stakeholders. It is an agency that accepts the reality that the environment causes risks to workers and is therefore worker friendly and knowledgeable about safety and toxic environments.[19] So if a different federal agency had been tasked with allocating post–9/11 funding, I think things would have been very different.

**Moline:** Though we are siloed in our distinct lines of work, the overarching objective was to find ways to go forward together. It would have been counterproductive to have one program combat the other. When David [Prezant] and I were grilled in the US Congress, for example, they asked us: "Why aren't you going to merge all the data together?" We said, "We can't do that. It's just not going to work," and we had to justify why scientifically. The complex, collaborative process with various groups on the ground and, ultimately, with the government, produced outcomes that saved lives.

**Siegel de Hernández:** Besides saving lives, advocacy improved the quality of lives and made a huge difference.

**Prezant:** Our work together, across groups, could not have existed without some degree of cooperation from all sides—in fact, unexpected amounts of cooperation—at different points in time and with different persons taking the lead. Sometimes it would be necessary for labor to push some buttons. Other times it was necessary for them to sit still and for management to push some buttons. And then it would flip again. And there were moments in time when that push needed to come from the community. That push wasn't orchestrated, it just happened. There were times when emotional advocacy is needed, and times when data-driven advocacy is needed. And the beauty of the WTC Health Program Steering Committee is that both have meshed. When we first went to Congress asking for money, the emotional advocacy got us in the door. But we weren't getting out the door because Congress kept saying, "There's no data. We don't believe this." It was the data that then allowed Congress to realize, through additional advocacy, that there was post–9/11 disease.

**Reibman:** To build on what David [Prezant] is saying about collaborations: David and I are nuanced and fact-based in our statements. We qualify our comments. We do not stand up and say something bluntly and dichotomously: "It's black and white." But you can't always do that as an advocate. So we've been learning and watching community members get up and say something with assurance to make a point and move a program forward. I'll never forget going to do a community presentation. I talked to one of the Beyond Ground Zero people who had been very friendly. And suddenly she got up and was lambasting me. But that was what you do as an advocate. You need to get a point across, and you don't worry about niceties and nuances. To understand that technique was a bit shocking. We physicians had to be educated about what it means to be an advocate. But the community also had to be educated about how to understand and work with medical and scientific information.

During a discussion with the WTC Health Registry about questions for a proposed survey, community members said, "We don't want it done that way, we want to do it a different way." Then we all met together and suggested, "Let's get educated about the language you are using so we can understand what you're saying and speak a similar language." 9/11 Environmental Action asked the New York City Department of Health to conduct the same epidemiology training they give to staff, but this time specifically for community members. The NYC DOH agreed. That was very unusual—you see that in some other groups, like WE ACT[20]—it has to do with language: Who speaks what language and how do you speak together? Advocacy efforts have to be long-term, and this program has had a lot of endurance.

*4. The Importance of Preparedness*

**Prezant:** We have to be able and ready to deal with the aftereffects of a next disaster. For example, after an initial rescue effort is over—whether that is seven, ten, twelve, or twenty-one days; there is controversy about the exact number—you're moving into the cleanup phase. That is when there is no excuse for exposing people to a hazardous environment. In the aftermath, how do you operationalize postdisaster safety? Immediately after the 1995 Oklahoma City bombings, the hazardous environment by successfully controlled by keeping people offsite. But this happened only by accident. Because it was believed that there was another bomb, five or ten blocks were fenced off. But if a dirty bomb had gone off in that area, there would be huge negativity about fencing off an area as large as would be needed.

I was on the Environmental Protection Agency panel for the cleanup of the World Trade Center site. Lot of mistakes were made. We now have a better picture of what would be needed to do health monitoring and health treatment, but a challenge that still remains for another disaster would be to prevent the kind of exposures we had after 9/11.

**Mejia:** The reality is that when you consider lessons learned, we know what the lessons are. The problem is trying to get others to understand what those lessons are. How do you prepare for another incident and how do you coordinate the various city agencies? If the Department of Environmental Protection is going to send a subject matter expert if it involves water or sewage, the appropriate city agency now has to train a member of my union, District Council 37, how to suit up and how to respond. But if you ask a city manager, "Have you trained staff and provided them with the equipment they need?" The answer is "No, we can't do that. We don't have the money."

So a lesson learned is that we need to train all the workers who are going to respond, including those who are going to be converted to first responders. If anything was learned, it is that many workers are needed for a major disaster and not just those who wear a uniform. So every New York City agency has to have a trained and equipped workforce that is ready to be deployed. If we cannot get that kind of commitment and cooperation, we're going to have the same difficult circumstances for future disasters.

**Siegel de Hernández:** There are many ways to be prepared. Preparedness is something we do in our health and safety work. For my union I know that Communications Workers of America[21] union members will be part of every disaster response. What you do not want to do is wait for the next disaster to start thinking about preparedness. We need to think through: What kind of training is needed? What kind of personal protective equipment? How do you get the resources? This is planning that could and should be done ahead of time. Our union has done that with some employers since 9/11, but there is still much work that needs to be done.

One of the tenets of responding to an emergency—particularly one with chemical or other hazards—is that when you don't have all the information about the hazards, you assume a higher level of protection until you have done a more detailed assessment to figure out whether or not you can gear down to a lower level of protection. In other words, protect people first. You can apply the precautionary principle to any kind of disaster providing there is sufficient preparedness and resources. Therefore, rushing in first without protections and then attempting to prove that there is an exposure problem later does not work because by then you have people exposed. That is backward. Then, if you find out how bad things are, it is too late because the harm has been done. We can and certainly should proactively protect workers who respond to emergencies.

## 5. The Importance of Tenacity

**Moline:** We have described some of our struggles, but it is also important to know that we are also optimistic. If you had asked any of us thirteen or fifteen years ago whether, in 2015, the US Congress would extend the Zadroga 9/11 Health and Compensation Act[22] that gave coverage to those afflicted with Ground Zero–related health issues for the next seventy-five years at a cost estimated at $7 billion, it would have seemed absolutely unlikely. But it did happen. Yes, there is always a struggle, and there will be continued struggles. We'll come together for those too. We have to have had some optimism to get this far.

**Crane:** Tenacity, tenacity, tenacity.

**Moline:** Yes, tenacity and optimism. The tenacity is there because we are still here working on these issues, and there is now a seventy-five-year continuation of the Zadroga Act.[23]

**Siegel de Hernández:** While we each were working on various things, there were a lot of things we came together on. And over time those groups formed a very large coalition. The medical professionals here don't just treat patients; they are also advocates for the programs that care for people.

**Prezant:** We know how to advocate for a patient, we know how to advocate for the small programs that we are responsible for. The community came together on this. These were exposed people, many had almost no medical background, and they taught themselves how to organize and be effective advocates. Labor organizers served their members just as physicians served their patients. Did those groups have all the tools and knowledge necessary to do this? No, they did not, nor had they done something this massive from a health perspective before. But they had more understanding of these issues on the ground than any of us.

**Siegel de Hernández**: Nobody handed us money. Nobody said, "Oh here.... Let's create these programs." Every single thing that exists right now to address 9/11 health problems exists because of all the people and groups, including sick responders and survivors, labor unions, community and other advocacy organizations, elected officials, even celebrities, who fought to get those resources and also to get the recognition that emerging health conditions were 9/11-related.

**Moline:** When we look back at the challenges of the past years, a lot has been overcome, and a lot remains to be done. We've all become greyer and more wrinkled and more cynical and more optimistic at the same time about what people can do and how hard it is to get there. There is value in continued advocacy in whatever way one can do it— whether it is by representing groups of workers in unions, representing groups of patients in medical departments, advocating for health and well-being as management and university faculty, or advocating as healthcare providers. There is much value in the ongoing efforts of folks in the community who stepped up and did a magnificent job in the face of absolute denial from external forces.

**Reibman:** We have been working together for almost sixteen years. And that means that you had people who were really advocates—not instant, do-it-while-it's-trendy advocates—but long-term, consistent advocates. That is unusual. This is not a "do it while it's hot" topic, and then they move on to advocate for something else. These are people who have been here for almost sixteen years. We know each other's wrinkles.

## Implications for Other Times and Places

**Prezant:** The one advantage that we had that not all environmental issues have is that the health sequelae after September 11 resulted from an attack on this country. That was the single most important thing that we were able to use. If you look at the environmental disasters that are happening throughout this country, for example, the reports of lead poisoning in Flint, Michigan, in 2015 did not get the attention that was warranted.

**Flynn:** I'm from New Orleans, Louisiana, and my mother and brother were in her apartment building during Hurricane Katrina in 2005. All of us in this group were watching in horror as that failed disaster response unfolded. The federal resources needed were not brought to bear—before or after—and more than 1,830 people died, including people who died in their attics waiting for rescue two days after the levees broke, flooding four-fifths of the city. What we also learned after Hurricane Katrina is that affected residents were left on their own to deal with their flood- and storm-damaged homes with very little guidance on how to protect themselves. Watching that, we had a sinking déjà vu feeling.

In the early stages of our post–9/11 struggle, we were incredibly lucky to have access to experts who volunteered to help shape community demands to the government. They legitimated our concerns and helped to arm us with a technical and scientific vocabulary. This was critical because when we went forth and we, the community, said, "These are hazardous conditions," the press response was, "On what authority can you say that?" Our doctors also embraced an advocacy role that was absolutely crucial to getting federal recognition for 9/11 community health impacts and the funding for the World Trade Center Health Program. And we are all beholden to the New York State Congressional Delegation for advocating for us at the federal level.

When I look at the post–Hurricane Katrina environmental advocates in Louisiana, and when I look at the environmentalists who advocate for folks who live in Cancer Alley,[24] they are operating in an intensely antiregulatory climate. They cannot so readily turn to their elected officials and say, "We think that the EPA needs to step up enforcement here" and get support for the kinds of action they need. We're seeing the same lack of support from the Michigan governor and his administration in the Flint lead poisoning disaster in 2015.[25]

When the BP oil spill happened in 2010, and the Gulf Coast community said that residents and workers were starting to have health effects—those going out in vessels, those working onshore to clean up the oil with no protective gear, and those who were living in shoreline communities – they were all getting Corexit oil dispersant blown into their faces twenty-four hours a day[26]—they didn't have anybody like our congressional representative, Jerry Nadler, to turn to. I take my hat off to the Louisiana advocates who have an uphill battle with no end in sight . . . and now, the research is showing that they were right about the harmful effects of the dispersant. Every day I am thankful that ultimately, here in New York, many of our elected officials were alert to the ongoing health emergency and fought to support our cause, protecting the health of those who were exposed to the WTC disaster.[27]

**Roberto Lucchini**: The knowledge that is available today from all this work together is very important. I understand the frustration and all the sadness that we have because of all that has happened. But, to be positive, all the knowledge that has ensued is important. I keep thinking of my conversation with Brussels public safety officials after the March 22, 2016, bombing of their subway and airport.[28] When you are there at the onset of trauma, you are faced with something huge, and it is important to know exactly what is important. The programs that we are discussing created critical knowledge.

## Epilogue: Emerging and Ongoing Issues

According to Dr. David Prezant, codirector for the Fire Department of the City of New York (FDNY) World Trade Center Medical Monitoring Program, health issues in the aftermath of the 9/11 attack included "almost all lung diseases, almost all cancers—such as issues of the upper airways, gastroesophageal acid reflux disease, post-traumatic stress, anxiety, panic and adjustment disorders."[29] This epilogue describes two emerging issues that grow of out this history: children's health after 9/11 and representations of post–9/11 health challenges in the 9/11 Memorial Museum.

### Children's Health After 9/11: Community Concerns

People exposed to toxic environmental conditions after 9/11 included the 35,000 children who resided in Lower Manhattan as well as the thousands of children from other New York City neighborhoods who attended Lower Manhattan schools.[30] Despite these numbers and the well-documented vulnerability of children to harm from toxic exposures, there has been little attention to the physical health impacts of the 9/11 disaster on this population. Environmental health risks to children were initially ignored or denied. There are now an increasing number of studies on 9/11 mental health impacts for children living in New York City, but little on how the World Trade Center disaster affected their physical health.

An October 2008 report by the New York City Health Department's WTC Health Registry found that post–9/11 asthma prevalence in children under five years of age who lived or attended school in Lower Manhattan was double the already high rate in the northeastern United States.[31] A handful of studies have documented respiratory[32] and neurodevelopmental[33] impacts, with the latter found in children exposed to WTC pollution prenatally.[34]

Community calls for a more systematic investigation of the physical health of the WTC-exposed children were ignored over many years. Parents had sought care from their own pediatricians for children with post–911 health issues long before the Bloomberg administration created the WTC Environmental Health Center (WTC EHC). In 2008, the WTC EHC opened its doors to affected children. To advise parents that specialized treatment was available for their children at the WTC EHC, 9/11 Environmental Action spearheaded a "Dear Parents" letters to households of students attending public schools in 2007 followed with a "mass backpack" letter to downtown middle school parents. WTC EHC's pediatric program grew to some three hundred children.

Following passage of the Zadroga Act in 2011, the Survivors Steering Committee, created to advise the WTC Health Program,[35] advocated prioritizing research on children's post–9/11 physical health; funding research on biologically plausible health effects of 9/11; and recognizing the exceptional nature of "disaster science," since no predisaster baseline data exist.[36] Research has recently found elevated cardiovascular risks in the exposed children, demonstrating the need for long-term follow-up studies.[37]

In 2018, the WTC EHC is treating 1,500 young adults exposed to the 9/11 disaster as children. Many children have now aged into the WTC Health Registry's adult cohort, though there has been attrition, on top of the already small number of children originally enrolled in the Registry in 2003–2004. Arguing that the cohort size and disproportionate affluence of those registered renders it insufficiently representative of the population of exposed children, the SSC called for exploring the feasibility of creating a new larger and more diverse cohort composed of students attending schools in the disaster area in the fall of 2001.

The challenge of enrolling a population of rapidly dispersing young adults is daunting, since most have graduated from public schools. But it is increasingly clear to researchers and policymakers that an evidence-based understanding of the health effects on disaster-impacted children is important and therefore a worthwhile investment.

*Representations of Post–9/11 Health in the September 11 Memorial Museum*

In May 2014, several members of the World Trade Center Survivors Steering Committee (SSC) visited the September 11 Memorial Museum, a preview offered to the 9/11 community, those directly touched by 9/11 who were not part of its curatorial process.[38] The last section of the museum's Historical Exhibition,[39] entitled "After 9/11," included narrative panels with text, photographs, and memorabilia recounting the struggle for recognition of 9/11-related environmental illnesses and federally funded monitoring and treatment of those affected.

SSC visitors found that the information conveyed was minimal, disjointed, and demeaning. For example, text referred to people who have suffered ill health as "those with health conditions claimed to be related to the World Trade Center disaster," insinuating that such claims were dubious despite the large and growing medical literature documenting the serious health issues linked to WTC toxic exposures. Indeed, more than 82,190 people were being monitored or receiving treatment at the WTC Health Program as of September 2017, and of this total, 1,442 have died.[40]

Labor-based stakeholders reached out to Manhattan Borough President Gale Brewer to request that she establish a committee to plan a monument dedicated to people who had lost their health or lives as a result of exposure to WTC toxins. In June 2014 Manhattan Borough President Brewer convened the Committee to Establish a Monument to 9/11 Responders and Survivors with a representative group of responders and survivors, US Congressman Jerry Nadler, and other elected officials. Following a robust discussion, she summarized the emerging consensus in a December 2014 letter to New York State Governor Andrew Cuomo, asking him to urge the Port Authority of New York and New Jersey to provide a "site of tribute and healing" at Ground Zero to raise public awareness of the "quiet and devastating" 9/11 health crisis and to honor the many who are sick and "whose sacrifice has been hidden."

On August 8, 2014, Kimberly Flynn and James Melius, who respectively chaired the Steering Committees of WTC Survivors and Responders, wrote the museum's president, Joe Daniels, expressing serious concerns about the exhibit's revisionist history of the government's mishandling of the 9/11 environmental disaster and language that casts doubt on the still-unfolding, well-documented health consequences of 9/11. The chairs noted that statements such as "After 9/11, the US government and New York City officials were criticized for allegedly not providing timely and accurate information about air quality in Lower Manhattan," undermined well-established facts about the federal government's failure to warn lower Manhattan workers and residents about environmental toxins.[41] "These errors," Flynn and Melius wrote, "obscure the truth about the causal link between WTC exposures and disease, and undermine federal efforts to provide all those whose health was harmed by 9/11 with specialized health care." They called on Daniels to correct text panels raising doubts about the causal connection between toxic exposures, a call reiterated in the *Daily News*.[42] The Museum revised the panels but nothing else in the "After 9/11" exhibit despite a meeting, described as productive, between the museum officials and labor and responder representatives.

In September 2016, the fifteenth anniversary of 9/11, Governor Cuomo announced that a monument would be built at Ground Zero "to pay tribute to the heroes who lost their lives, as well as those survivors who continue to suffer from health issues related to the aftermath of the terrorist attack."[43] Further negotiations resulted in a May 30, 2017, announcement that the museum would take the lead in "the planning, design and development of the dedication, with the Memorial's architects, including Michael Arad," with the tribute funded jointly by New York State and Bloomberg Philanthropies, headed by former New York City Mayor Michael Bloomberg.[44]

The Museum set the date for a stakeholders' meeting on July 14, 2017. However, the meeting did not include representatives from the survivor community or the Manhattan Borough President's Office, which had moved this initiative forward. The Museum's lack of inclusivity drew objections from the responder community, 9/11 family members, and 9/11 Museum Board member Jon Stewart.

The meeting's upshot was a "homework assignment": to respond in writing to questions of who or what should be honored in the tribute and what the tribute should achieve. The SSC joined other groups in submitting responses, reflecting the stakeholder consensus by calling on the Museum to establish "a meaningful and substantial structure to honor all responders and survivors who have lost their health or their lives due to exposures to the toxic aftermath of the destruction of the World Trade Center."

The Museum's "2017 Year in Review" blog entry mentioned the proposed memorial that would "recognize the courage and sacrifice of rescue and recovery workers and to honor all those who are suffering or have died from 9/11-related illnesses."[45] Stakeholders expected a follow-up meeting at the Museum to provide an update and gather further input from representatives of all constituencies, but at the time of this writing, such a meeting has yet to be announced.

## Appendix A: Bionotes—Introductions at the Beginning of the April 6, 2016, Meeting

**Michael Crane**, M.D., medical director for the World Trade Center Health Program (for responders) at Mt. Sinai

I'm the medical director for the Sinai clinic for the World Trade Center Health Program. We are a responder clinic, so we see rescue and recovery workers. At the time of 9/11, I was a medical director for Con Edison. I experienced firsthand the whole time and I saw a lot of workers down there—thousands of them, actually. I became interested in the impact on them because I saw it. When I had the opportunity, I came up to Sinai and started working there. I'm still here.

**Kimberly Flynn**, cofounder of 9/11 Environmental Action; Chair of the WTC Health Program Survivor Steering Committee

I'm a cofounder of 9/11 Environmental Action, a key 9/11 advocacy organization, and have been the chair or co-chair of the WTC Health Program's Survivors Steering Committee for more than five years. My earliest involvement was helping to organize the community in the vicinity of the World Trade Center site in the fall of 2001. In April 2002, 9/11 Environmental Action formed as a coalition that would pursue protective action. We held an environmental summit that brought together Lower Manhattan residents, school parents and occupational safety and environmental health advocates who united behind an effort to press the Environmental Protection Agency for proper testing and cleanup of World Trade Center (WTC) indoor contamination from homes, schools and workplaces. As it became clear that health impacts were emerging in the community—the same impacts that were emerging in the responder population—we worked with Dr. Reibman and with another coalition called the Beyond Ground Zero Network, which was largely Chinatown and Lower East Side based. 9/11EA, BGZ, and other community and labor groups advocated strongly for the community to be included in the Zadroga bill. We formed an advisory body, which is a precursor to the WTC Health Program's Survivors Steering Committee. This is the counterpart to the Responders Steering Committee—both were created under the Zadroga Act to represent the two WTC-exposed populations, survivors and responders, respectively.

**Roberto Lucchini,** M.D., director, Mt Sinai Division of Occupational and Environmental Medicine

I am the director of the data center at Mount Sinai. I was not in New York, nor in this country, on 9/11. I was in Italy, where I have been working in occupational medicine for many years. I came to the program at Mt. Sinai and to New York in 2012. My interest in this program is constantly growing. Knowledge of this program is limited outside the United States. So I have put as much effort as possible into sharing knowledge from the program and what is done here. This program can provide important knowledge to those in Europe and elsewhere.

**Guille Mejia,** MPH, CHES; Safety & Health Director, Safety & Health Department, District Council 37, AFSCME, AFL-CIO

I am the director of the Safety and Health Department of District Council 37, American Federation of State, County and Municipal Employees (AFSCME). District Council 37 is a labor organization representing city, state and cultural workers Many of our members responded to 9/11 and performed a variety of tasks at Ground Zero and the surrounding areas as well as the landfill. Our members were there from day one and continued to be present at the site until it was turned over to private contractors. DC 37 represents both the uniformed EMS personnel as well as non-uniformed personnel at various city agencies who did a lot of work post 9/11 and had many kinds of exposures. Initially and right after 9/11, I worked on getting the city to protect our members from the safety and health hazards they were encountering and then on getting proper medical help for those injured and exposed to the toxic environments. To this day, my staff and I continue to do outreach and protect our members' interests.

**Jacqueline Moline,** M.D., Hofstra Northwell School of Medicine; vice president of Occupational Medicine, Epidemiology and Prevention; founding chair of Population Health/Occupational Medicine, Epidemiology and Prevention for the new Hofstra Northwell School of Medicine

I am currently at Northwell Health involved in the Queens World Trade Center Clinical Center. Prior to that, I was at Mount Sinai and was one of the founders of the WTC responder program. We started seeing patients in our occupational medical center within the first two to three weeks. We were seeing people who needed treatment. We began a concerted effort working closely with organized labor. We spearheaded it with Senator Clinton to get initial funding for the program, which was obtained mid-April 2002. Then, we started seeing patients three months later. There was a lot of work done in three months to staff a clinical center and start the programs that have evolved into a multicenter of excellence program. Then, it morphed in 2006 when we began to treat patients with federal dollars as opposed to using philanthropy—which had kept many of the treatment programs going in the early years. I had continued involvement. And then I directed the program at Mount Sinai before I left for my new position in 2010.

**Cristina Onea**, doctoral student, The Graduate Center, City University of New York

I am a PhD student at the CUNY Graduate Center in Critical Social and Personality Psychology. My interests are in surveillance and the effects of surveillance on social relationships and trust.

**Susan Opotow**, PhD, John Jay College of Criminal Justice and The Graduate Center, City University of New York

I am a City University of New York professor and a social psychologist, and I am on the sociology faculty at John Jay College of Criminal Justice and head the PhD Program in Critical Social/Personality Psychology at the Graduate Center. My research is on the psychology of conflict and justice. After 9/11 I saw these issues arise repeatedly in larger and smaller ways. I wanted to pull together a book that would track how key issues after 9/11 unfolded over time in New York City. This kind of book could be helpful to people who lived through 9/11, and it could also help us all better understand how the aftereffects of 9/11 unfolded over time.

**David Prezant**, M.D., chief medical officer and codirector of the World Trade Center Health Program, Fire Department of New York City

I'm the chief medical officer for the New York City Fire Department, special advisor to the Fire Commissioner on health policy, and codirector of the World Trade Center and Medical Monitoring Program. I think what Micki Siegel de Hernández is talking about is the really central mission that, in any other disease, people know the disease exists. People are doing research on why the disease occurs and what would be the best treatment. It's already covered by Medicare and health insurance companies. It's a process that keeps on going, thankfully, in this country that for most people—unfortunately not for all—but for many people, they have access to that. This was different. This put people in a position that they were not used to being in. We're not used to being environmental scientists who are advocates for research scientists and large groups of people.

**Joan Reibman**, M.D., medical director of the World Trade Center Survivor Program

I'm a medical director of the World Trade Center survivor program. I've been working with health in the community since early on. My focus has really been on World Trade Center's adverse health effects in the local community.

**Micki Siegel de Hernández,** MPH, health and safety director, Communications Workers of America, District 1

I am the health and safety director for the Communications Workers of America (CWA) here in the Northeast. CWA represents members in many different occupations. We had thousands of members who were responders, members who were survivors, as well as members who died on that day. We have been involved since that time, initially dealing with employers for the members that we represented, but also—from the very beginning—working with the occupational health community because it was clear that there were contaminants and it wasn't unexpected that there would be health problems that would result. People were symptomatic from very early on. From 9/11 forward, this has been a continuous process. The work has been done around these issues on a daily basis. You also can't separate out the health issues and the programs that have developed, from the advocacy that was needed in order to get there. It was hard enough on the responders' side. First, we had the Fire Department when David Prezant and others sounded the alarm. Then, it was recognition that other response workers who were also exposed were getting sick. And the hardest battle was for the survivor community.

## Notes

*The authors are listed alphabetically, so that the first and second authors are not necessarily the primary ones.

1. Nordgrén, Goldstein, and Izeman, 2002.

2. Prezant, Weiden, Banauch, McGuinness, Rom, Aldrich, and Kelly, 2002; Moline, Herbert, Crowley, Troy, Hodgman, Shukla, Udasin et al., 2009.

3. "What We Know about the Health Effects of 9/11: A Message from the Commissioner of the New York City Department of Health and Mental Hygiene," https://goo.gl/yH6DGG; Nordqvist, 2011; Justin Worland, "Health Problems Linger for 9/11 First Responders," *Time*, April 16, 2015.

4. Reibman, Levy-Carrick, Miles, Flynn, Hughes, Crane, and Lucchini, 2016; Crane, Levy-Carrick, Crowley, Barnhart, Dudas, Onuoha, Globina, Haile, Shukla, and Ozbay, 2014.

5. Newman, 2013.

6. Thomas R. Frieden (MD, MPH) became the director of the Centers for Disease Control and Prevention and administrator of the Agency for Toxic Substances and Disease Registry on June 8, 2009.

7. *"Ground Zero"* referred to the World Trade Center site after the 9/11 attacks.

8. See Newman, 2013, 8–10.

9. See Lederman et al., 2004.

10. Laurie Garrett is a science journalist who wrote "I Heard the Sirens Scream."

11. Sheldon Silver was a Democratic Party politician from New York City who rose to become the powerful Speaker of the New York State Assembly from 1994 to 2015.

12. See Newman, 2013.

13. Anthony DePalma, "Judge Dismisses 9/11 Suit Against Former Head of E.P.A.," *New York Times*, April 23, 2008.

14. See https://goo.gl/gUfVgD.

15. Crane et al., 2014.

16. The American Federation of Labor and Congress of Industrial Organizations (AFL-CIO) is the largest federation of unions in the United States.

17. A *dirty bomb* is a weapon used to spread radioactive material with conventional explosives.

18. There were several community coalitions, including BGZ, 9/11EA and the WTC Community-Labor Coalition. Kimberly Flynn comments (personal communication, November 2016): "What the community lacked was an institutional infrastructure, something that labor had."

19. See https://goo.gl/XZtHNm.

20. WE ACT for Environmental Justice—Empowering Communities to Power Change is an environmental, community-driven, political-change organization in West Harlem, New York City. See https://goo.gl/A8E3ez.

21. CWA members work in telecommunications and information technology, the airline industry, news media, broadcast and cable television, education, health care, public service, law enforcement, manufacturing, and other fields. See https://goo.gl/GR5DCT.

22. James L. Zadroga was a New York City police officer who was a first responder. He died of a respiratory disease attributed to his participation as a rescue worker at Ground Zero.

23. For information on the James L. Zadroga 9/11 Health & Compensation Act, see https://goo.gl/MTCCms.

24. Cancer Alley, Louisiana. See https://goo.gl/3HNU5o.

25. Yanan Wang, "In Flint, Mich., There's So Much Lead in Children's Blood That a State of Emergency Is Declared," *Washington Post*, December 15, 2015.

26. From the Center for Biological Diversity: "BP used two dispersants called Corexit 9500A and Corexit 9527A . . . Dispersants are chemicals that are sprayed on a surface oil slick to break down the oil into smaller droplets that more readily mix with the water." See https://goo.gl/YADfth.

27. Dispersants can turn oil spills into toxic mist, research shows. *Times-Picayune*, March 21, 2018. See https://goo.gl/wGoRtj.

28. Victoria Shannon, "Brussels Attacks: What We Know and Don't Know," *New York Times*, March 22, 2016.

29. Leah McGrath Goodman, "9/11's Second Wave: Cancer and Other Disease Linked to the 2001 Attacks are Surging," *Newsweek*, September 16, 2016.

30. Based on the US Year 2000 Census, 35,000 children eighteen years old and under resided below 14th Street in Manhattan. See https://goo.gl/7foQqZ.

31. Stellman, Thomas, Osahan, Brackbill, and Farfel, 2013.

32. Thomas, Brackbill, Thalji, DiGrande, Campolucci, Thorpe, and Henning, 2008.

33. Lederman, Rauh, Weiss, Stein, Hoepner, Becker, and Perera, 2004.

34. See Columbia Center for Environmental Health: https://goo.gl/s7MG2n.

35. The SSC advocates for the needs of survivors with health impacts of 9/11. Its members include representatives of community-based organizations, advocacy organizations, and labor groups that serve this population as well as individuals exposed to environmental contaminants released as a result of the attack on the WTC. See https://goo.gl/YVXmj9.

36. See https://goo.gl/drALrV.

37. Trasande, Koshy, Gilbert, Burdine, Marmor, Han, Shao, Chemtob, Attina, and Urbina, 2018.

38. See Greg B. Smith, "9/11 Memorial and Museum Will Open for Families of Victims, First Responders after Anniversary Ceremony," *New York Daily News*, September 9, 2014.

39. The Historical Exhibition, located within the original footprint of the North Tower of the World Trade Center, tells the story of 9/11 using artifacts, images, first-person testimony, and archival audio and video recordings. The exhibition is made up of three sequential parts: the Events of the Day, Before 9/11, and After 9/11.

40. See the World Trade Center (WTC) Health Program, Program Statistics, September 30, 2017, available at https://goo.gl/7Q3oT5.

41. Nordgrén, Goldstein, and Izeman, 2002.

42. Dan Friedman, "Anger Over 9/11 Museum Exhibit that Casts Doubt on Link between Health Problems and Toxic Ground Zero Air," *New York Daily News*, August 10, 2014; Editorial, "The Truth and Nothing But: 9/11 Museum Must Correct Exhibits on Ground Zero Air Toxins," *New York Daily News*, August 14, 2014.

43. "Governor Cuomo Announces Monument to be Built Honoring 9/11 First Responders and Survivors: State Will Launch Request for Proposals to Select Design and Location for Monument in New York City," New York State, September 11, 2016, available at https://goo.gl/igQt2n; Glenn Blain, "Ground Zero Recovery Workers to Be Honored with Their Own Monument at 9/11 Memorial," *New York Daily News*, May 31, 2017.

44. "Governor Cuomo and Mayor Bloomberg Announce Planning of a

Permanent Dedication to Ground Zero Rescue and Recovery Workers at the 9/11 Memorial," May 30, 2017. https://goo.gl/xQVy4o.

45. *"Year in Review: 2017 at the 9/11 Memorial & Museum," December 29, 2017.* https://goo.gl/8gRmT2.

## References

Crane, Michael A., Nomi C. Levy-Carrick, Laura Crowley, Stephanie Barnhart, Melissa Dudas, Uchechukwu Onuoha, Yelena Globina, Winta Haile, Gauri Shukla, and Fatih Ozbay. "The Response to September 11: A Disaster Case Study." *Annals of Global Health* 80, no. 4 (2014): 320–331.

Lederman, Sally Ann, Virginia Rauh, Lisa Weiss, Janet L. Stein, Lori A. Hoepner, Mark Becker, and Frederica P. Perera. "The Effects of the World Trade Center Event on Birth Outcomes among Term Deliveries at Three Lower Manhattan Hospitals." *Environmental Health Perspectives* 112, no. 17 (2004): 1772.

Moline, Jacqueline M., Robin Herbert, Laura Crowley, Kevin Troy, Erica Hodgman, Gauri Shukla, Iris Udasin, et al. "Multiple Myeloma in World Trade Center Responders: A Case Series." *Journal of Occupational and Environmental Medicine* 51, no. 8 (2009): 896–902.

Newman, David M. "Protecting Worker and Community Health: Are We Prepared for the Next 9/11?" New York, NY: New York Committee for Occupational Safety and Health (NYCOSH). December 30, 2013.

Nordgrén, Megan D., Eric A. Goldstein, and Mark A. Izeman. *The Environmental Impacts of the World Trade Center Attacks: A Preliminary Assessment.* Washington, DC: Natural Resources Defense Council, 2002.

Nordqvist, C. "9/11 Ten Years On: The Health Effects on Rescue Workers." https://goo.gl/2T8nUd.

Prezant, David J., Michael Weiden, Gisela I. Banauch, Georgeann McGuinness, William N. Rom, Thomas K. Aldrich, and Kerry J. Kelly. "Cough and Bronchial Responsiveness in Firefighters at the World Trade Center Site." *New England Journal of Medicine* 347, no. 11 (2002): 806–815.

Reibman, Joan, Nomi Levy-Carrick, Terry Miles, Kimberly Flynn, Catherine Hughes, Michael Crane, and Roberto G. Lucchini. "Destruction of the World Trade Center Towers: Lessons Learned from an Environmental Health Disaster." *Annals of the American Thoracic Society* 13, no. 5 (2016): 577–583.

Stellman, Steven D., Pauline A. Thomas, Sukhminder S. Osahan, Robert M. Brackbill, and Mark R. Farfel. "Respiratory Health of 985 Children Exposed to the World Trade Center Disaster: Report on World Trade Center Health Registry Wave 2 Follow-up, 2007–2008." *Journal of Asthma* 50, no. 4 (2013): 354–363.

Thomas, Pauline A., Robert Brackbill, Lisa Thalji, Laura DiGrande, Sharon Campolucci, Lorna Thorpe, and Kelly Henning. "Respiratory and Other

Health Effects Reported in Children Exposed to the World Trade Center Disaster of 11 September 2001." *Environmental Health Perspectives* 116, no. 10 (2008): 1383.

Trasande, Leonardo, Tony T. Koshy, Joseph Gilbert, Lauren K. Burdine, Michael Marmor, Xiaoxia Han, Yongzhao Shao, Claude Chemtob, Teresa M. Attina, and Elaine M. Urbina. "Cardiometabolic Profiles of Adolescents and Young Adults Exposed to the World Trade Center Disaster." *Environmental Research* 160 (2018): 107–114.

# Posttraumatic Stress Disorder Following 9/11
## What We Know Now

Ari Lowell, Ariel Durosky, Anne Hilburn,
Liat Helpman, Xi Zhu, and Yuval Neria

I see it all again, sometimes. Every day, at least once. Once I stopped sleeping, it got much harder. Actually I can't remember when I stopped totally being able to sleep. I sleep two hours a night. At first it was different, now—I toss and turn all night, it's awful. I can't think or concentrate at all. I am terribly irritable. Got in a fistfight yesterday with someone who was winding me up. I suddenly snapped. I'm not like this. I've never been this way before. I could always sleep it off; my nickname is _____. I feel like I'm going crazy inside. I have these panic attacks. I don't want to be dramatic but it feels like I'm going to die. I have felt stress before. But nothing ever like this.[1]

The preceding quotation is taken from an article summarizing findings from narratives of trauma exposure by rescue and recovery workers who were present directly following the events of the September 11 attacks on the World Trade Center. The ramifications of a terrorist attack of the magnitude of 9/11 across emotional, social, and political spectrums are exceedingly widespread,[2] and the specific damage in terms of economic cost, loss of life, and injury is unlike any other terrorist attack in US history.[3] But these aspects tell only part of the story; as the preceding description illustrates, a key component of the devastation caused by 9/11 is its impact on mental health. Among mental health problems that develop following a large-scale traumatic event, posttraumatic stress disorder (PTSD) is the most common consequence.[4]

180

This chapter outlines what we have learned regarding the prevalence of PTSD among those directly exposed to 9/11 and how the expression of PTSD may change over time. Some of the critical questions this chapter addresses include: how high were rates of PTSD following 9/11? Who was most at risk? What risk factors contributed to the development of PTSD? And finally, what have we learned in recent years that advances our knowledge and perceptions formed by earlier research?

## PTSD

PTSD is defined as a maladaptive reaction to traumatic stress. An event is considered "traumatic" in the clinical sense if it involves significant threat to life, serious injury, or sexual assault.[5] Trauma exposure may also involve witnessing a significant threat to another person, learning about the traumatic experience of a close family member or friend, or experiencing repeated exposure to details of a traumatic event. Some examples in the context of 9/11 include watching another person jump from the World Trade Center (WTC) and assisting in the recovery of human remains. Although most who undergo trauma exposure successfully integrate these experiences without ill effects, for a subset of individuals, such traumatic memories cause life difficulties that may affect a person's relationships, ability to work, and overall well-being.

PTSD is distinguished by four hallmark features. The first is intrusive thoughts or reexperiencing symptoms. Intrusive thoughts occur when a person thinks about the traumatic event frequently in a way that causes distress and has difficulty dismissing such thoughts. Intrusive thoughts can take the form of nightmares or "flashbacks," which are the realistic sensations associated with reliving the traumatic experience. The rescue worker exhibits reexperiencing symptoms in the cited example when he says, "I see it all again, sometimes. Every day, at least once."

A second feature of PTSD is avoidance of trauma reminders. Because remembering the traumatic event is so distressing, and because reminders of this event can trigger an intense fear response, individuals with PTSD will often go to great lengths to avoid thinking or talking about their trauma. They may even avoid situations or stimuli that serve as reminders of what happened or that trigger memories connected with fear. Some signs of avoidance are more obvious, such as a person's unwillingness to return to the site of 9/11. But other signs are subtler, such as avoiding a family gathering where someone may be discussing 9/11, not wanting to be in other tall buildings, avoiding former coworkers from the WTC, and so forth. Avoidance symptoms often have a profound impact on life functioning by interfering with a person's capacity to work and socialize.

A third feature of PTSD, recently added to the formal diagnosis of this disorder, is negative changes in cognitions or mood. This includes difficulty remembering details of the traumatic event, loss of interest in previously enjoyed activities, feeling detached from others, and persistent negative feelings such as anger, guilt, and fear. Severe guilt can be a particularly distressing outcome of PTSD. For example, one 9/11 victim reported feeling intensely guilty for passing people during her rush to escape the towers, even though she herself struggled greatly to make it down the stairwell and nearly did not escape.[6] "Changes in cognitions" refers to marked change in beliefs about oneself, the world, and others, such as development of the notion that "the world is inherently unsafe" or "bad things are likely to happen to people at any time." Such thoughts can influence a person's behavior. In a treatment case study, for example, a patient described feeling especially vulnerable to attack, which led this patient to avoid riding the subway, eventually leading to her inability to work.[7] Other changes in beliefs may concern feeling damaged or inferior in some way, losing trust in others, or losing hope for the future.

The final feature of PTSD is hypervigilance and hyperarousal. Individuals with PTSD may be preoccupied by the idea of danger and engage in a constant state of alert. Physiological arousal is often heightened by "triggers" such as thoughts about a traumatic event or environmental stimuli such as particular sounds, smells, and sights. Indeed, a number of rescue workers referred to smells associated with their trauma exposure—as one said, "the smell of death everywhere."[8] Such individuals may also experience a rapid activation of the autonomic nervous system, the "fight-or-flight" response. Classic symptoms associated with hypervigilance/hyperarousal include irritability, constant scanning for danger, exaggerated startle response, concentration difficulties, and sleep disturbances.

Thus, PTSD can be a pervasive and highly disruptive disorder. Those who developed symptoms of PTSD following 9/11 have described severe impairment in work ability due to such problems as concentration difficulties, intense fear when travelling, disruption of personal relationships related to changes in mood, feelings of withdrawal and disconnection, feelings of panic, constant worry, alertness to danger, and intrusive thoughts related to watching people being injured and killed or handling human remains.[9]

Although the question of why some people develop this disorder and others do not is the subject of some debate, research has been helpful in determining risk factors that increase the likelihood of PTSD. A primary risk factor is severity of exposure.[10] As one might expect, more intensive and persistent trauma exposure is a predictor of PTSD.

## Previous Research

For the tenth anniversary of the attacks, we conducted a thorough review of research concerning the prevalence of PTSD in populations highly exposed to 9/11.[11] At that time we limited our research to "high exposure" populations (i.e., those in close proximity to the attacks or its aftermath) due to their higher risk of developing PTSD. Two important findings from our review were, first, that prevalence rates for PTSD were not consistent across high-exposure populations; and, second, PTSD symptoms gradually decreased for some groups, but not others. We also identified some of the major risk factors for the development and maintenance of PTSD as well as factors affecting resilience, recovery, and the development of other mental health problems.

Since this review was published, additional research has been conducted concerning those highly exposed to 9/11. Much data have been made available through several organized registries such as the World Trade Center Health Registry (WTCHR), which contains information on more than 71,000 people exposed to 9/11, and the World Trade Center Health Program (WTCHP), a treatment and monitoring program established to benefit survivors and rescue workers. Newer data includes more expansive longitudinal data describing the course of PTSD over time.

For this chapter, we expanded our earlier review of research on populations highly exposed to 9/11. We included articles previously reviewed and highlighted areas informed by more recent studies. In the process, we answer the questions we posed earlier regarding PTSD prevalence, the course of PTSD, and risk factors associated with PTSD.

## Methods

Our previous review surveyed reports on 9/11 highly exposed populations published between October 2001 and April 2011.[12] For the present chapter, we identified additional studies published between 2011 and May 2016, again focusing on those who have been highly exposed to 9/11. Table 1 provides a summary of studies conducted over the last 15 years since 9/11 ($n = 47$), emphasizing key data on prevalence rates and risk factors. New reports that did not appear in our previous review are marked

with an asterisk (*). We added tables summarizing prevalence rates across
both studies (Table 2) and the course of PTSD as per longitudinal studies
(Table 3).

## Findings

*Prevalence*

For studies previously reviewed, prevalence rates of probable PTSD during
the first year following 9/11 encompassed a wide range from as low as
1.5 percent to as high as 29.6 percent (see Table 2). One reason for the
high degree of variability among these studies is their focus on different
specific populations of interest, as some highly exposed populations were
prone to higher rates of PTSD than others. For example, rates of PTSD
were lower among community samples than among children and Pentagon staff. A high degree of variability was often present across articles
focusing on the same population as well, although some of this variability
may be explained by differences in measurement and sampling methods.
The smallest amount of within-group variability was present among first
responders and rescue workers, with estimates of this group's prevalence
rates centered closely around 10 percent.

Prevalence rates of PTSD collected during subsequent periods tended
to be lower, suggesting that overall rates of PTSD can be expected to fall
over time (see Table 2). However, this finding was not consistent across
all groups, and wide variability was again present. Data at later time periods was also very limited for some groups, such as children/adolescents.
Notably, while rates tended to fall over time among most groups, rates for
first responders/rescue workers collected after the first year saw a relative
increase compared to rates observed in other groups.

As may be expected, the majority of articles reviewed in our previous
study utilized data from between one and four years post–9/11. In contrast, most of the articles reviewed for this chapter collected data between
two to eleven years after 9/11, and nearly all solely concerned rescue/
recovery workers. We found no recent studies that examined prevalence
rates among children. As found previously, most of the more recent studies showed increasing rates of PTSD at later time points for rescue and
recovery workers, which again contrasted with decreasing rates among
other high-exposure populations. Prevalence rates from these more recent
studies also reflected a wide range (see Table 2). An important nuance
present across a number of studies in the more recent review was differ-

ences found between traditional (e.g., police, firemen) and nontraditional responders (e.g., utility workers, lay volunteers). Only two studies in our previous review considered nontraditional responders as an independent group, and only one compared these groups directly. In contrast, three of the present studies examined differences between traditional and nontraditional responders and two focused on nontraditional responders specifically. These studies, as well as the one study previously reviewed, all found higher rates of PTSD among nontraditional responders when compared to traditional responders (see Table 1 for details).

*The Course of PTSD*

As with prevalence rates, the course of PTSD varied greatly across populations. A relatively small number of longitudinal studies examining change over time were available at the time of our previous study, but most also showed a reduction in rates of PTSD across most populations (see Table 3). The exception again was for studies of rescue and recovery workers. In contrast to reductions in rates for other populations, rates for rescue and recovery workers tended to modestly increase over time, with only one study finding a very small decrease four years post–9/11.

We reviewed eight articles containing longitudinal data for this chapter (see Table 3). An advantage of these studies over those included in the previous review is that these studies generally spanned a longer period of time and were better able to utilize more comprehensive data from existing 9/11 registries, as discussed. One study of primary care patients found a reduction in PTSD of 6 percent over time, consistent with decreasing rates of PTSD for most populations. The remaining six studies focused on rescue and recovery workers. These studies again found rates of PTSD to increase over time for this population, although rates of PTSD appeared to increase more for traditional than for nontraditional responders, with two studies indicating that rates may have decreased for nontraditional responders at a later time point. An exception was one study that indicated increasing rates of PTSD among lay and affiliated volunteers, but particularly for lay volunteers; however, this study did not directly compare traditional and nontraditional responders.[13]

*Risk Factors*

Despite some inconsistencies and variability in the literature, our previous review found direct exposure to 9/11 as a clear predictor of PTSD, with loss of life of significant others, physical injury, and immediate risk of life following as additional prominent risk factors. Community samples included further risk factors such as female gender, younger or older age, low education/income, history of mental disorder, and belonging to an ethnic minority, whereas among studies of first responders/rescue workers, probable PTSD correlated with anger, depression, psychiatric distress, impaired social/occupational functioning, and psychiatric history (see Table 1).

Risk factors found in our present review were similar to those previously outlined, although again most of the present studies focused on rescue and recovery workers. Identified risk factors were severity of trauma exposure, traumatic loss, female gender, minority ethnicity, lower education, poor employment, lack of social integration, unmet health care needs, prior psychiatric diagnosis, and general life stress (see Table 1).

Notably, the availability of additional longitudinal data was helpful in further outlining risk factors for chronic PTSD in high exposure 9/11 populations. Some identified specific risk factors for chronic PTSD in a sample of police responders include recent life stressor, lower levels of social support, sustained injuries during 9/11, unmet mental health care needs, and female gender.[14] In contrast, symptom severity, trauma history, major depression, occupational exposure, and panic disorder were shown to predict PTSD chronicity in a sample of utility workers.[15] Social support at home and work was shown to have a possible protective effect among both traditional and nontraditional responders,[16] while ongoing stress occurring after 9/11 may inhibit PTSD recovery.[17] Significantly, several studies identified health-related unemployment as a particularly important risk factor for chronic PTSD.[18]

## Discussion

The purpose of this chapter was to explore questions about the prevalence, course, and associated risk factors of PTSD in high-exposure 9/11 populations, as well as to recap and update our previous review.[19] We also examined how more recent literature advanced existing knowledge. While many of the studies presently reviewed repeat and confirm earlier findings, a number contribute new information and serve to expand some areas of interest. In particular, several newer studies utilizing longitudinal data were helpful in further examining the course and development of PTSD, including chronic PTSD. Our current review also revealed some areas that were unexpectedly understudied and warrant additional attention.

As with our previous review, a clear answer regarding the prevalence of PTSD is confounded by a high degree of variability in studies across population of focus, time point of data collection, and methodology utilized, which is a limitation of these research findings. Nonetheless, we were able to distinguish a general trend consistent with earlier findings suggesting that rates of PTSD are highest for those with the greatest trauma exposure, and that these rates typically decrease over time. The exception was again for rates of rescue and recovery workers, which became more elevated. Two contributions of the present review were to highlight the continuation of this trend across a longer time period, and also to note differences between traditional and nontraditional responders.

One possible explanation for differences we found between traditional and nontraditional responders is that nontraditional responders receive less formal training and may also receive less support. An alternative explanation, which is supported by increasing incidence of PTSD over time in the first-responder population, is that traditional responders may be more reluctant to report initial symptoms or may otherwise utilize coping mechanisms that delay the effects of trauma until a later point in time. Certainly, resistance to seeking help among uniformed officers is well known.[20]

An additional contribution of the current chapter, which answers our initial question—how recent advances in the literature inform current knowledge and understanding—is that health-related unemployment secondary to an injury sustained during 9/11 was indicated as a strong risk factor for the development and maintenance of PTSD and especially for chronic PTSD. This risk factor is likely particularly disabling because it interferes with occupational and social activity, which have both been identified as protective factors. Such an injury may also serve to compound PTSD as a constant, debilitating reminder of the experienced trauma.

Although findings regarding rescue and recovery workers are exceedingly valuable, a lack of recent studies concerning other high exposure populations, especially children, was perhaps our most surprising finding. The absence of more child-focused studies is especially striking in light of organized efforts to provide treatment to affected children and adolescents in the wake of 9/11, such as by the Child and Adolescent Treatment Services (CATS) Consortium. This program collected data from approximately seven hundred children and adolescent participants across multiple treatment sites in formulating its recommendations for implementation for treatment for traumatized youth in the wake of a disaster.[21]

Table 1. Epidemiological Articles Concerning Posttraumatic Stress Disorder (PTSD) in Populations Highly Exposed to World Trade Center Attacks on September 11, 2011 (9/11)

| Source | Sample | Sample size | Time frame of data collection post 9/11 | PTSD prevalence estimate (%) | PTSD correlates |
|---|---|---|---|---|---|
| **Community or General Population** | | | | | |
| Adams & Boscarino, 2006 | NYC residents | 1,681 (71% of baseline sample) | 1 year, 2 years | 5.0, 3.8 | Year 1: Younger age, female gender, more 9/11 disaster events, more non–9/11 traumatic events, more negative life events, low social support, low self-esteem; Year 2: Middle age, Hispanic ethnicity, more post–9/11 traumas and negative life events, low self-esteem |
| DiGrande et al., 2008 | Lower Manhattan residents | 11,037 | 2–3 years | 12.5 | Older age, female gender, Hispanic ethnicity, low education and income, divorce, 9/11 events: injury, witnessing horror, and dust cloud exposure |
| Galea et al., 2002 | Manhattan residents | 1,008 | 5–8 weeks | 7.5 | Hispanic ethnicity, 2" prior stressors, panic attack near time of WTC attacks, residence south of Canal Street, event-related loss of possessions |
| Galea et al., 2003 | NYC residents | 2,752 | 4 months, 6 months | 2.3, 1.5 | Directly affected |
| Schlenger et al., 2002 | U.S. households, oversample in NYC and Washington, DC | 2,273 | 1–2 months | NYC = 11.2; Washington, DC = 2.7; other major metropolitan areas = 3.6; rest of United States = 4.0 | Female gender, younger age, direct exposure, amount of viewing 9/11 television coverage |

## Specific Populations
### First responders and/or rescue and recovery workers

| Study | Population | Sample | Time points | Prevalence | Correlates of higher numbers of PTS symptoms |
|---|---|---|---|---|---|
| Silver et al., 2005 | U.S. residents, some directly exposed in NYC and Washington, DC | 1,906 (75% of baseline sample) | 2 weeks, 1 year | Directly exposed = 9.3 Acute Stress Disorder (ASD) 11.2; exposed via live television = 12.8 (ASD), 4.7; no live exposure = 10.4 (ASD), 3.4 | Higher numbers of acute stress symptoms 2 weeks post–9/11, direct exposure, African American ethnicity, pre–9/11 diagnosis of mental disorder, low education |
| Berninger, Webber, Niles, et al., 2010 | Firefighters | 5,656 (83.3% of baseline sample) | 0–6 months, 3–4 years | 8.6, 11.1 | Impaired functioning |
| Berninger, Webber, Cohen, et al., 2010 | Firefighters | 10,074 total (8,679 at 1 year; retention of baseline sample: 10.8% at 2 years, 26.7% at 3 years, 40.3% at 4 years) | 1 year, 2 years, 3 years, 4 years | 9.8, 9.9, 11.7, 10.6 | Earliest arrival at site, prolonged work at site, supervising on site without prior supervisory experience, retirement due to 9/11-related disability, impaired functioning at home and work |
| *Bowler et al., 2012 | Police responders | 2,940 | 2–3 years, 5–6 years | 7.8, 16.5 | Female gender (at time 1 but not time 2), disability, loss of job post-9/11 |
| *Bromet et al., 2016 | WTC responders | 3,231 | 11–13 | 9.7 | Exposure severity, physical health, life satisfaction |
| Chiu et al., 2011 | Retired firefighters | 1,915 | 4–6 years | 22.0 | Earlier arrival at site |
| *Cone et al., 2015 | Police responders | 2,204 | 2–3 years, 5–8 years, 10–11 years | 4.8, 11.9, 11 | Older age at exposure, recent life stressors, unmet mental health needs, lower social support, injuries, female gender |

*(continued)*

Table 1. (*continued*)

| Source | Sample | Sample size | Time frame of data collection post 9/11 | PTSD prevalence estimate (%) | PTSD correlates |
|---|---|---|---|---|---|
| Cukor, Wyka, Jayasinghe, et al., 2011 | Utility workers | 2,960 | 10–34 months | 8 | Psychiatric or trauma history, subjective perception of threat to one's life, higher exposure to the site |
| *Cukor, Wyka, Mello, et al., 2011 | Utility workers | 1,983 | 1–2 years, 3–4 years, 6–7 years | PCL: 9.5, 4.8, 2.4; CAPS: 14.9, 8.4, 5.8 | MDD 1–2 years post–9/11, higher 9/11 exposure, prior trauma history, panic disorder |
| *Debchoudhury et al., 2011 | Volunteer disaster recovery workers (affiliated and lay) | 4,974 | 2–3 years, 5–8 years | Lay: 20.2, 29.6; Affiliated: 7.5, 11.2 | Lay volunteer vs. affiliated volunteer status |
| Evans, Giosan, Patt, Spielman, & Difede, 2006 | Disaster relief workers | 626 | 21–25 months | 5.8 | Anger, distress, reduced social and occupational functioning |
| Evans, Patt, Giosan, Spielman, & Difede, 2009 | Utility workers | 842 | 17–27 months | 5.9 | Impaired social and occupational functioning, history of trauma, history of panic disorder or depression |
| Jayasinghe, Giosan, Evans, Spielman, & Difede, 2008 | Disaster relief workers | 1,040 | 3 years | 6.8 | Anger, depression, psychiatric distress |

| Study | Population | Sample size | Time frame | Rate (%) | Risk factors/findings |
|---|---|---|---|---|---|
| *Luft et al., 2012 | Police responders and nontraditional responders | 8,508 police, 12,333 nontraditional | 1–7 years | 5.9 (police responders), 23 (nontraditional responders) | Nontraditional responder vs. police responder, PTSD associated with higher rates of respiratory distress |
| Perrin et al., 2007 | Rescue and recovery workers | 28,962 | 2–3 years | 12.4 | Job type (higher rates in construction, engineering, and sanitation workers), being an unaffiliated volunteer, earlier start date (except for police), longer duration of time worked at site (except for police), performing tasks not common to one's occupation |
| *Pietrzak et al., 2014 | Police responders and nontraditional responders | 4,035 police, 6,800 nontraditional | 3, 6, and 8 years (average time frames) | Police: 8.5, 9.3, 9.8; Nontraditional: 24.1, 24.2, 22.5 | Hispanic ethnicity, psychiatric diagnosis prior to 9/11, more pre–9/11 stressors, higher exposure to the site, 9/11-related medical conditions, older age |
| *Pietrzak et al., 2012 | Police responders | 8,466 | 1–7 years | 5.4 | Low social support, more pre–9/11 stressors, older age, knowing someone who was killed or injured in the attacks |
| Stellman et al., 2008 | Rescue and recovery workers | 10,132 | 10–61 months | 11.1 | Impaired social functioning, loss of family member or friend in the attacks, disruption of family, work, and social life, behavioral symptoms in workers' children |
| *Webber et al., 2011 | Firefighters and EMS workers | 10,867 | 6–9 years | 6.9 | Early arrival and length of exposure to WTC site |

*(continued)*

Table 1. (*continued*)

| Source | Sample | Sample size | Time frame of data collection post 9/11 | PTSD prevalence estimate (%) | PTSD correlates |
|---|---|---|---|---|---|
| *Yip et al., 2015 | EMS workers | 2,281 | Up to 12 years post–9/11 | 7 | Early arrival to WTC site |
| *Zvolensky et al., 2015 | Rescue and recovery workers | 8,466 police and 10,430 nontraditional | 1–9 years V1, V2 completed average of 2.5 years following V1 | V1: 11.7 for police, 16.4 for nontraditional responders; V2: 13 for police, 17.2 for nontraditional responders | Level of exposure, stressful events post 9/11, demographic factors |
| **Pentagon staff** | | | | | |
| Grieger, Fullerton, & Ursano, 2003 | Pentagon staff | 77 | 7 months | 14.0 | Higher initial emotional response, higher peritraumatic dissociation, female gender, lower perceived safety 7 months post–9/11 |
| Grieger, Fullerton, & Ursano, 2004 | Pentagon staff | 212 | 13 months | 23.0 | Direct exposure, lower perceived safety 13 months post–9/11 at home and work, and in usual activities and |
| Grieger, Waldrep, Lovasz, & Ursano, 2005 | Pentagon staff | 267 | 25 months | 16.0 | At Pentagon on 9/11, sustaining injury, witnessing dead bodies, acting as lay counselor to families of the deceased |
| Jordan et al., 2004 | Pentagon staff | 1,837 | 1–4 months | 7.9 | Reduced daily functioning, less use of counseling services |

## World Trade Center evacuees

| | | | |
|---|---|---|---|
| DiGrande, Neria, Brackbill, Pulliam, & Galea, 2011 | WTC towers evacuees | 3,271 | 2–3 years | 15.0 | Female gender, minority racial identity, lower income, direct exposure (i.e., higher floor in towers, later evacuation, caught in dust cloud after collapses of towers, witnessing horror, sustaining injury), working for an employer who was killed in the attacks |

## New York City workers

| | | | |
|---|---|---|---|
| Tapp et al., 2005 | NYC transit workers | 269 | 7.5 months | 8.0 | Exposure to the dust cloud after collapses of towers |
| Thiel de Bocanegra, Moskalenko, & Kramer, 2006 | NYC Chinatown workers | 148 | 28 months | 42.0 | Higher post–9/11 likelihood of visiting physician, receiving prescription drugs, or indicating interest in counseling |

## Primary care patients

| | | | |
|---|---|---|---|
| Neria, Gross, & Marshall, 2006 | Manhattan primary care patients | 930 | 7–16 months | 4.7 | At baseline, approximately 1 year after 9/11, PTSD was associated with Hispanic ethnicity, being born outside of the US, not being married, pre–9/11 family psychiatric history, and pre–9/11 trauma; in addition, PTSD was found to be associated with comorbid mental disorder, impaired functioning, and increased use of mental health medication |

*(continued)*

Table 1. (*continued*)

| Source | Sample | Sample size | Time frame of data collection post 9/11 | PTSD prevalence estimate (%) | PTSD correlates |
|---|---|---|---|---|---|
| Neria et al., 2008 | Bereaved primary care patients | 252 | 7–16 months | 17.1 | Knowing someone who was killed in the attacks |
| Neria et al., 2010 | Manhattan primary care patients | 455 (46% of baseline sample) | 1 year, 4 years | 9.6, 4.1 | Overall: pre–9/11 major depressive disorder, impaired functioning. Follow-up: major depressive and anxiety disorders |
| *Neria et al., 2013 | Primary care patients with direct, indirect exposure, or 9/11 related bereavement | 444 | 1 year, 4 years | 10, 4 | Direct exposure, knowing someone who was killed in the attacks |
| **Mixed adult samples** | | | | | |
| Brackbill et al., 2009 | Rescue and recovery workers, lower Manhattan residents and office workers, passersby | 43,032 (subsample of 46,322 [68.1% of baseline sample] assessed for asthma) | 2–3 years, 5–6 years | 14.3, 19.1 | Wave 2 (5–6 years): 9/11—related loss of spouse or job, eligibility group (higher rate in passersby) |
| *Caramanica, Brackbill, Liao, & Stellman, 2014 | Rescue and recovery workers, lower Manhattan residents, and office workers, passersby | 29,486 | 10–11 years | 15.20 | Higher 9/11 exposure, health-related unemployment, poorer outcomes on employment measures, lack of social integration, lower quality of life, perceived unmet mental health care needs. |

| Study | Sample | N | Time since | % | Risk/associated factors |
|---|---|---|---|---|---|
| Farfel et al., 2008 | Building occupants, people on street or in transit in Lower Manhattan on 9/11, local residents, rescue and recovery workers and volunteers, school children and staff | 68,444 | 2–3 years | 16.3 | Hispanic ethnicity, household income below $25,000, sustaining injury |
| **Children and adolescents** | | | | | |
| Brown & Goodman, 2005 | Children with WTC parent death | 49 | $M = 10.5$ months | 20.4 | Traumatic grief |
| DeVoe, Klein, Bannon, & Miranda Julian, 2011 | NYC children 0–5 years old | 180 | 9–13 months | 14.0 | Direct exposure, trauma history, negative changes in parenting, increased tension between parents |
| Fairbrother, Stuber, Galea, Fleischman, & Pfefferbaum, 2003 | NYC children 4–7 years old | 434 | 4–5 months | 18.0 | Parental PTSD, parent crying in front of child, seeing 3" graphic images of the disaster on television, Manhattan residence |
| Hoven et al., 2005 | NYC public schoolchildren | 8,236 | 6 months | 10.6 | Higher exposure, female gender, lower grade level, exposure of family member, trauma history |

(continued)

Table 1. (*continued*)

| Source | Sample | Sample size | Time frame of data collection post 9/11 | PTSD prevalence estimate (%) | PTSD correlates |
|--------|--------|-------------|------------------------------------------|------------------------------|-----------------|
| Mullett-Hume, Anshel, Guevara, & Cloitre, 2008 | Chinatown middle school children | 204 | 2.5 years | 35.0 | Higher numbers of non–9/11–related traumas |
| Pfeffer, Altemus, Heo, & Jiang, 2007 | Children with WTC parent death | 79 (retention not reported) | 4 months–2 years (time of study entry varied) | 29.6 at 4 months, gradual decline to 5 at 2 years | Hypothalamic–pituitary adrenal axis dysregulation |
| Rosen & Cohen, 2010 | NYC public schoolchildren | 7,832 | 6 months | 7.4–26.8 | Lower grade level, direct exposure of family member or friend |

Table 2. Summary of prevalence rates of PTSD by number of years assessed post–9/11

| Population (number of studies) | First year range | 2 to 4 year range | 4 to 8 year range | 8+ year range |
|---|---|---|---|---|
| *Previous review (rates presented as %)* | | | | |
| Community or general population (3,2) | 1.5–11.2 | 3.8–12.5 | — | — |
| First responders and/or rescue and recovery workers (2,8,1) | 8.6–14.9 | 4.8–12.4 | 22 | — |
| Pentagon Staff (3,1) | 7.9–23 | 16 | — | — |
| World Trade Center evacuees (2) | — | 15 | — | — |
| New York City workers (1,1) | 8 | 42 | — | — |
| Primary care patients (3,1) | 4.7–17.1 | 4.1 | — | — |
| Mixed adult samples (2,1) | — | 14.3–16.3 | 19.1 | — |
| Children and adolescents (6,2) | 7.4–29.6 | 5–35 | — | — |
| Overall (18,19,2) | 1.5–29.6 | 3.8–42 | 19.1–22 | — |
| *Present review (rates presented as %)* | | | | |
| First responders and/or rescue and recovery workers (4,4,4)[a] | — | 4.8–24.1 | 5.4–29.6 | 2.4–22.5 |
| Primary care patients (1) | 10 | 4 | — | — |
| Mixed adult samples (1) | — | — | — | 15.2 |
| Overall (1,3,3,4) | 10 | 4–24.1 | 5.4–24.2 | 2.4–22.5 |

[a] Five studies did not differentiate between data collected between the first and subsequent years. Time collection for these studies cumulatively ranged between 10 months and nine years after 9/11. Prevalence rates for these studies ranged from 5.9 percent to 23 percent.

A lack of follow-up regarding findings and data therefore represents a significant missed opportunity that lacks a clear explanation, though an absence of funding, long-term planning, and interest are possible factors. The lack of data on youth also suggests the need for appropriate planning for long-term studies in children and adolescents following natural or man-made disasters in the future, along with additional efforts to examine the effects of treatment. Such data would also provide more detailed information about the long-term effectiveness of specific treatment interventions.

The present findings have implications for policy. First, knowledge of which populations are most affected by trauma, which risk factors are associated with PTSD, and how PTSD develops over time in different groups is critically important for treatment and intervention planning. Knowing that traditional responders are likely to report initial lower rates of PTSD but higher subsequent symptomatology, for example, can guide intervention specialists to target care and consider barriers to treatment, such as fear of mental-health stigma. Likewise, knowledge of risk factors is especially important in directing preventative care. It may also be helpful to strengthen such protective factors as social and occupational support, particularly for vulnerable populations. This approach may especially benefit nontraditional responders who may experience a relatively high degree of exposure but may have a less supportive framework. Specific knowledge of the effects of injury on mental health in the aftermath of a mass tragedy is also critical in order to provide such individuals with adequate care and attention.

Second, our research illustrates the usefulness of central health registries. Such registries may serve as an important tool for collecting data on those affected by large-scale disasters. They can track initial rates of disorders, the course of illness, and risk/protective factors over time. Centralized registries carry the added benefit of using consistent measurement tools, which may reduce the high variability noted across both our reviews. These registries would do well to include all high-exposure populations, and not just particular groups (such as first responders) as occurred following 9/11. Youth in particular represent a population that was well studied within the first year following 9/11 but subsequently failed to attract sufficient empirical attention.

In sum, this chapter provides important information regarding rates of PTSD over time for populations with the greatest exposure to the events of 9/11, especially rescue and recovery workers. PTSD is a highly disabling condition, and knowledge about how people are affected and who is most at risk is critical to the mustering appropriate resources for treatment and support. What we have learned, however, also highlights what we do not know: how specific populations, particularly children and ordinary civilians, may become and remain affected in the many years since 2001. We hope these findings will inform policy related to the anticipated risk for PTSD and will inspire the development of appropriate responses. These findings underscore the need for the collection of longitudinal data across all affected highly exposed populations in advance of the unfortunate circumstance of future disasters, man-made or natural.

Table 3. Measured changes in prevalence of PTSD by population as reported by longitudinal studies

| Population | Approximate time between data collections | Percent change (%) |
|---|---|---|
| | *Previous review* | |
| Community or general population | | |
|   Adams & Boscarino, 2006 | 1 year | −1.2 |
|   Silver et al., 2005 | 2 years | −1.2 |
| First responders and/or rescue and recovery workers | | |
|   Berninger, Webber, Cohen, et al., 2010 | Data collected at 1 year intervals over four time points | +.1, +1.8, −1.1 |
|   Berninger, Webber, Niles, et al., 2010 | 3–4 years | +2.5 |
| Primary care patients | | |
|   Neria et al., 2010 | 3 years | −5.5 |
| Mixed adult samples | | |
|   Brackbill et al., 2009 | 3–4 years | −4.8 |
| Children and adolescents | | |
|   Pfeffer, Altemus, Heo, & Jiang, 2007 | 2 years | −24.6 |
| | *Present review* | |
| First responders and/or rescue and recovery workers | | |
|   Bowler et al., 2012[a] | 3–4 years | +8.7 |
|   Cone et al., 2015[a] | Data collected at 2–3 year intervals over three time points | +7.1, −.9 |
|   Cukor, Wyka, Mello, et al., 2011[b] | 1–3 years, 3–4 years | PCL: −4.7, −2.4; CAPS: −6.5, −2.6 |
|   Debchoudhury et al., 2011 | 3–6 years | Affiliated volunteers: +3.7; Lay volunteers: +9.4 |
|   Pietrzak et al., 2014 | Data collected at 2–3 year intervals over three time points | Police: +.8, +.5; Nontraditional responders: +.1, −1.7 |
|   Zvolensky et al., 2015 | 2.5 years | Police: +1.3; Nontraditional responders: +.8 |
| Primary care patients | | |
|   Neria et al., 2013 | 2–4 years | −6 |

[a] Sample consisted of traditional responders only.

[b] Sample consisted of nontraditional responders only.

## Notes

1. Bills et al., 2009, 186.
2. Comer and Kendall, 2007.
3. Kunreuther, Michel-Kerjan, and Porter, 2003.
4. Breslau et al., 1998.
5. American Psychiatric Association, 2013.
6. Kazi, Freund, and Ironson, 2008.
7. Difede and Eskra, 2002.
8. Bills et al., 2009, 183.
9. Ibid.; Katz et al., 2006.
10. Neria, DiGrande, and Adams, 2011.
11. Ibid.
12. Ibid.
13. Cukor et al., 2011.
14. Cone et al., 2015.
15. Cukor et al., 2011.
16. Pietrzak et al., 2014.
17. Zvolensky et al., 2015.
18. Bowler et al., 2012; Caramanica et al., 2014; Pietrzak et al., 2014.
19. Neria, DiGrande, and Adams, 2011.
20. Steinkopf, Hakala, and Van Hasselt, 2015.
21. Costantino et al., 2014.

## References

Adams, Richard E., and Joseph A. Boscarino. "Predictors of PTSD and Delayed PTSD after Disaster: The Impact of Exposure and Psychosocial Resources." *Journal of Nervous and Mental Disease* 194, no. 7 (2006): 485–493.

American Psychiatric Association. *Diagnostic and Statistical Manual of Mental Disorders : DSM–5*. Washington, DC: American Psychiatric Association, 2013.

Berninger, Amy, Mayris P. Webber, Hillel W. Cohen, Jackson Gustave, Roy Lee, Justin K. Niles, Sydney Chiu, et al. "Trends of Elevated PTSD Risk in Firefighters Exposed to the World Trade Center Disaster: 2001–2005." *Public Health Reports* 125, no. 4 (2010): 556–566.

Berninger, Amy, Mayris P. Webber, Justin K. Niles, Jackson Gustave, Roy Lee, Hillel W. Cohen, Kerry Kelly, Malachy Corrigan, and David J. Prezant. "Longitudinal Study of Probable Post-Traumatic Stress Disorder in Firefighters Exposed to the World Trade Center Disaster." *American Journal of Industrial Medicine* 53, no. 12 (2010): 1177–1185.

Bills, Corey B., Nancy Dodson, Jeanne M. Stellman, Steven Southwick, Vansh Sharma, Robin Herbert, Jacqueline M. Moline, and Craig L. Katz. "Stories Behind the Symptoms: A Qualitative Analysis of the Narratives of 9/11

Rescue and Recovery Workers." *Psychiatric Quarterly* 80, no. 3 (2009): 173–189.

Bocanegra, Heike Thiel, Sophia Moskalenko, and Elizabeth J. Kramer. "PTSD, Depression, Prescription Drug Use, and Health Care Utilization of Chinese Workers Affected by the WTC Attacks." *Journal of Immigrant and Minority Health/Center for Minority Public Health* 8, no. 6 (2006): 203–210.

Bowler, Rosemarie M., Matthew Harris, Jiehui Li, Vihra Gocheva, Steven D. Stellman, Katherine Wilson, and Howard Alper. "Longitudinal Mental Health Impact among Police Responders to the 9/11 Terrorist Attack." *American Journal of Industrial Medicine* 55 (2012): 297–312.

Brackbill, Robert M., James L. Hadler, Laura DiGrande, Christine C. Ekenga, Mark R. Farfel, Stephen Friedman, Sharon E. Perlman, et al. "Asthma and Posttraumatic Stress Symptoms 5 to 6 Years Following Exposure to the World Trade Center Terrorist Attack." *Journal of the American Medical Association* 302, no. 5 (2009): 502–516.

Breslau, N., R. C. Kessler, H. D. Chilcoat, L. R. Schultz, G. C. Davis, and P. Andreski. "Trauma and Posttraumatic Stress Disorder in the Community: The 1996 Detroit Area Survey of Trauma." *Archives of General Psychiatry* 55, no. 7 (1998): 626–632.

Bromet, E. J., M. J. Hobbs, S. A. P. Clouston, A. Gonzalez, R. Kotov, and B. J. Luft. "DSM-IV Post-Traumatic Stress Disorder among World Trade Center Responders 11–13 Years after the Disaster of 11 September 2001 (9/11)." *Psychological Medicine* 46, no. 4 (2016): 771–783.

Brown, Elissa J., and Robin F. Goodman. "Childhood Traumatic Grief: An Exploration of the Construct in Children Bereaved on September 11." *Journal of Clinical Child and Adolescent Psychology* 34, no. 2 (2005): 248–259.

Caramanica, Kimberly, Robert M. Brackbill, Tim Liao, and Steven D. Stellman. "Comorbidity of 9/11-Related PTSD and Depression in the World Trade Center Health Registry 10–11 Years Postdisaster." *Journal of Traumatic Stress* 27, no. 6 (2014): 680–688.

Chiu, Sydney, Mayris P. Webber, Rachel Zeig-Owens, Jackson Gustave, Roy Lee, Kerry J. Kelly, Linda Rizzotto, et al. "Performance Characteristics of the PTSD Checklist in Retired Firefighters Exposed to the World Trade Center Disaster." *Annals of Clinical Psychiatry* 23, no. 2 (2011): 95–104.

Comer, Jonathan S., and Philip C. Kendall. "Terrorism: The Psychological Impact on Youth." *Clinical Psychology: Science and Practice* 14, no. 3 (2007): 179–212.

Cone, James E., Jiehui Li, Erica Kornblith, Vihra Gocheva, Steven D. Stellman, Annum Shaikh, Ralf Schwarzer, and Rosemarie M. Bowler. "Chronic Probable PTSD in Police Responders in the World Trade Center Health Registry Ten to Eleven Years after 9/11." *American Journal of Industrial Medicine* 493 (2015): 483–493.

Costantino, Giuseppe, Louis H Primavera, Robert G Malgady, and Erminia Costantino. "Culturally Oriented Trauma Treatments for Latino Children Post 9/11." *Journal of Child and Adolescent Trauma* 7, no. 4 (2014): 247–255.

Cukor, Judith, Katarzyna Wyka, Brittany Mello, Megan Olden, Nimali Jayasinghe, and Jennifer Roberts. "The Longitudinal Course of PTSD among Disaster Worker Deployed to the World Trade Center Following the Attacks of September 11th." *Journal of Traumatic Stress* 24, no. 5 (2011): 506–514.

Debchoudhury, Indira, Alice E. Welch, Monique A. Fairclough, James E. Cone, Robert M. Brackbill, Steven D. Stellman, and Mark R. Farfel. "Comparison of Health Outcomes among Affiliated and Lay Disaster Volunteers Enrolled in the World Trade Center Health Registry." *Preventive Medicine* 53, no. 6 (2011): 359–363.

DeVoe, Ellen R., Tovah P. Klein, William Bannon, and Claudia Miranda-Julian. "Young Children in the Aftermath of the World Trade Center Attacks." *Psychological Trauma: Theory, Research, Practice, and Policy* 3, no. 1 (2011): 1–7.

Difede, JoAnn, and David Eskra. "Cognitive Processing Therapy for PTSD in a Survivor of the World Trade Center Bombing." *Journal of Trauma Practice* 1, no. 3–4 (2002): 155–165.

DiGrande, Laura, Y. Neria, R. M. Brackbill, P. Pulliam, and S. Galea. "Long-Term Posttraumatic Stress Symptoms Among 3,271 Civilian Survivors of the September 11, 2001, Terrorist Attacks on the World Trade Center." *American Journal of Epidemiology* 173, no. 3 (2011): 271–281.

DiGrande, Laura, Megan A. Perrin, Lorna E. Thorpe, Lisa Thalji, Joseph Murphy, David Wu, Mark Farfel, and Robert M Brackbill. "Posttraumatic Stress Symptoms, PTSD, and Risk Factors among Lower Manhattan Residents 2–3 Years after the September 11, 2001 Terrorist Attacks." *Journal of Traumatic Stress* 21, no. 3 (2008): 264–273.

Evans, Susan, Cezar Giosan, Ivy Patt, Lisa Spielman, and JoAnn Difede. "Anger and Its Association to Distress and Social/occupational Functioning in Symptomatic Disaster Relief Workers Responding to the September 11, 2001, World Trade Center Disaster." *Journal of Traumatic Stress* 19, no. 1 (2006): 147–152.

Evans, Susan, I. Patt, E. Giosan, L. Spielman, and J. Difede. "Disability and Posttraumatic Stress Disorder in Disaster Relief Workers Responding to September 11, 2001, World Trade Center Disaster." *Journal of Clinical Psychology* 65, no. 7 (2009): 684–694.

Fairbrother, Gerry, Jennifer Stuber, Sandro Galea, Alan R. Fleischman, and Betty Pfefferbaum. "Posttraumatic Stress Reactions in New York City Children after the September 11, 2001, Terrorist Attacks." *Ambulatory Pediatrics* 3, no. 6 (2003): 304–311.

Farfel, Mark, Laura DiGrande, Robert Brackbill, Angela Prann, James Cone, Stephen Friedman, Deborah J. Walker, et al. "An Overview of 9/11 Experiences and Respiratory and Mental Health Conditions among World Trade Center Health Registry Enrollees." *Journal of Urban Health* 85, no. 6 (2008): 880–909.

Galea, Sandro, Jennifer Ahern, Heidi Resnick, Dean Kilpatrick, Michael Bucuvalas, Joel Gold, and David Vlahov. "Psychological Sequelae of the September 11 Terrorist Attacks in New York City." *New England Journal of Medicine* 346, no. 13 (2002): 828–833.

Galea, Sandro, David Vlahov, Heidi Resnick, Jennifer Ahern, Ezra Susser, Joel Gold, Michael Bucuvalas, and Dean Kilpatrick. "Trends of Probable Post-Traumatic Stress Disorder in New York City after the September 11 Terrorist Attacks." *American Journal of Epidemiology* 158, no. 6 (2003): 514–524.

Grieger, Thomas A., Carol S. Fullerton, and Robert J. Ursano. "Posttraumatic Stress Disorder, Alcohol Use, and Perceived Safety after the Terrorist Attack on the Pentagon." *Psychiatric Services* 54, no. 10 (2003): 1380–1382.

———. "Posttraumatic Stress Disorder, Depression, and Perceived Safety 13 Months after September 11." *Psychiatric Services* 55, no. 9 (2004): 1061–1063.

Grieger, Thomas A., Douglas A. Waldrep, Monica M. Lovasz, and Robert J. Ursano. "Follow-up of Pentagon Employees Two Years after the Terrorist Attack of September 11, 2001." *Psychiatric Services* 56, no. 11 (2005): 1374–1378.

Hoven, C. W., C. S. Duarte, C. P. Lucas, P. Wu, D. J. Mandell, R. D. Goodwin, M. Cohen, et al. "Psychopathology among New York City Public School Children 6 Months after September 11." *Archives of General Psychiatry* 62, no. 5 (2005): 545–552.

Jayasinghe, Nimali, Cezar Giosan, Susan Evans, Lisa Spielman, and JoAnn Difede. "Anger and Posttraumatic Stress Disorder in Disaster Relief Workers Exposed to the September 11, 2001 World Trade Center Disaster: One-Year Follow-up Study." *The Journal of Nervous and Mental Disease* 196, no. 11 (2008): 844–846.

Jordan, Nikki N., Charles W. Hoge, Steven K. Tobler, James Wells, George J. Dydek, and Walter E. Egerton. "Mental Health Impact of 9/11 Pentagon Attack: Validation of a Rapid Assessment Tool." *American Journal of Preventive Medicine* 26, no. 4 (2004): 284–293.

Katz, C. L., R. Smith, M. Silverton, A. Holmes, C. Bravo, K. Jones, M. Kiliman, et al. "Open Forum: A Mental Health Program for Ground Zero Rescue and Recovery Workers: Cases and Observations." *Psychiatric Services* 57, no. 9 (2006): 1335–1338.

Kazi, A., B. Freund, and G. Ironson. "Prolonged Exposure Treatment for Posttraumatic Stress Disorder Following the 9/11 Attack with a Person Who Escaped from the Twin Towers." *Clinical Case Studies* 7, no. 2 (2008): 100–117.

Kunreuther, Howard, Erwann Michel-Kerjan, and Beverly Porter. "Assessing, Managing, and Financing Extreme Events: Dealing with Terrorism." National Bureau of Economic Research, December 22, 2003. https://goo.gl/T1tJ5K.

Luft, B. J., C. Schechter, R. Kotov, J. Broihier, D. Reissman, K. Guerrera, I. Udasin, et al. "Exposure, Probable PTSD and Lower Respiratory Illness among

World Trade Center Rescue, Recovery and Clean-up Workers." *Psychological Medicine* 42, no. 5 (2012): 1069–1079.

Mullet-Hume, E., D. Anshel, V. Guevara, and M. Cloitre. "Cumulative Trauma and Posttraumatic Stress Disorder among Children Exposed to the 9/11 World Trade Center Attack." *American Journal of Orthopsychiatry* 78 (2008): 103–108.

Neria, Yuval, Laura DiGrande, and Ben G. Adams. "Posttraumatic Stress Disorder Following the September 11, 2001, Terrorist Attacks: A Review of the Literature among Highly Exposed Populations." *American Psychologist* 66, no. 6 (2011): 429–446.

Neria, Yuval, Raz Gross, Mark Olfson, Marc J. Gameroff, Priya Wickramaratne, Amar Das, Daniel Pilowsky, et al. 2006. "Posttraumatic Stress Disorder in Primary Care One Year after the 9/11 Attacks." *General Hospital Psychiatry* 28, no. 3 (2006): 213–222.

Neria, Yuval, Mark Olfson, Marc J. Gameroff, Laura DiGrande, Priya Wickramaratne, Raz Gross, Daniel J. Pilowsky, et al. 2010. "Long-Term Course of Probable PTSD after the 9/11 Attacks: A Study in Urban Primary Care." *Journal of Traumatic Stress* 23, no. 4 (2010): 474–482.

Neria, Yuval, Mark Olfson, Marc J. Gameroff, Priya Wickramaratne, Raz Gross, Daniel J. Pilowsky, Carlos Blanco, et al. "The Mental Health Consequences of Disaster-Related Loss: Findings from Primary Care One Year after the 9/11 Terrorist Attacks." *Psychiatry* 71, no. 4 (2008): 339–348.

Neria, Yuval, Priya Wickramaratne, Mark Olfson, Marc J. Gameroff, Daniel J. Pilowsky, Rafael Lantigua, Steven Shea, and Myrna M. Weissman. "Mental and Physical Health Consequences of the September 11, 2001 (9/11) Attacks in Primary Care: A Longitudinal Study." *Journal of Traumatic Stress* 26, no. 1 (2013): 45–55.

Perrin, Megan A., Laura Digrande, Katherine Wheeler, and Lorna Thorpe. "Differences in PTSD Prevalence and Associated Risk Factors Among World Trade Center Disaster Rescue and Recovery Workers." *American Journal of Psychiatry* 164 (2007): 1385–1394.

Pfeffer, Cynthia R., Margaret Altemus, Moonseong Heo, and Hong Jiang. "Salivary Cortisol and Psychopathology in Children Bereaved by the September 11, 2001, Terror Attacks." *Biological Psychiatry* 61, no. 8 (2007): 957–965.

Pietrzak, Robert H., A. Feder, R. Singh, C. B. Schechter, E. J. Bromet, C. L. Katz, D. B. Reissman, et al. "Trajectories of PTSD Risk and Resilience in World Trade Center Responders: An 8-Year Prospective Cohort Study." *Psychological Medicine* 44, no. 1 (2014): 205–219.

Pietrzak, Robert H, Risë B. Goldstein, Steven M. Southwick, and Bridget F. Grant. "Physical Health Conditions Associated with Posttraumatic Stress Disorder in U.S. Older Adults: Results from Wave 2 of the National Epidemiologic Survey on Alcohol and Related Conditions." *Journal of the American Geriatrics Society* 60, no. 2 (2012): 296–303.

Rosen, C. S., and M. Cohen. "Subgroups of New York City Children at High Risk of PTSD after the September 11 Attacks: A Signal Detection Analysis." *Psychiatric Services* 61, no. 1 (2010): 64–69.

Schlenger, William E., Juesta M. Caddell, Lori Ebert, B. Kathleen Jordan, Kathryn M. Rourke, David Wilson, Lisa Thalji, J. Michael Dennis, John a. Fairbank, and Richard A. Kulka. 2002. "Psychological Reactions to Terrorist Attacks." *Journal of the American Medical Association* 288, no. 5 (2002): 581.

Silver, Roxane Cohen, E. Alison Holman, Daniel N. McIntosh, Michael Poulin, Virginia Gil-Rivas, and Judith Pizarro. "Coping with a National Trauma: A Nationwide Longitudinal Study of Responses to the Terrorist Attacks of September 11th." In *9/11: Mental Health in the Wake of Terrorist Attacks*, edited by Yuval Neria, Raz Gross, and Randall Marshall, 45–70. New York: Cambridge University Press, 2005.

Steinkopf, Bryan L., Kori A. Hakala, and Vincent B. Van Hasselt. "Motivational Interviewing: Improving the Delivery of Psychological Services to Law Enforcement." *Professional Psychology: Research and Practice* 46, no. 5 (2015): 348–354.

Stellman, Jeanne Mager, Rebecca P. Smith, Craig L. Katz, Vansh Sharma, Dennis S. Charney, Robin Herbert, Jacqueline Moline, et al. "Enduring Mental Health Morbidity and Social Function Impairment in World Trade Center Rescue, Recovery, and Cleanup Workers: The Psychological Dimension of an Environmental Health Disaster." *Environmental Health Perspectives* 116, no. 9 (2008): 1248–1253.

Tapp, Loren C., Sherry Baron, Bruce Bernard, Richard Driscoll, Charles Mueller, and Ken Wallingford. "Physical and Mental Health Symptoms among NYC Transit Workers Seven and One-Half Months after the WTC Attacks." *American Journal of Industrial Medicine* 47, no. 6 (2005): 475–483.

Webber, Mayris P., Michelle S. Glaser, Jessica Weakley, Jackie Soo, Fen Ye, Rachel Zeig-Owens, Michael D. Weiden, et al. "Physician-Diagnosed Respiratory Conditions and Mental Health Symptoms 7-9 Years Following the World Trade Center Disaster." *American Journal of Industrial Medicine* 54, no. 9 (2011): 661–671.

Yip, Jennifer, Rachel Zeig-Owens, Mayris P. Webber, Andrea Kablanian, Charles B. Hall, Madeline Vossbrinck, Xiaoxue Liu, et al. "World Trade Center–Related Physical and Mental Health Burden among New York City Fire Department Emergency Medical Service Workers." *Occupational and Environmental Medicine* (2015): 1 9.

Zvolensky, Michael J., Roman Kotov, Clyde B. Schechter, Adam Gonzalez, Anka Vujanovic, Robert H Pietrzak, Michael Crane, et al. "Post-Disaster Stressful Life Events and WTC-Related Posttraumatic Stress, Depressive Symptoms, and Overall Functioning among Responders to the World Trade Center Disaster." *Journal of Psychiatric Research* 61 (2015): 97–105.

# Living in Houses Without Walls
## Muslim Youth in New York City in the Aftermath of 9/11

### Diala Shamas

I felt like I was living in a house without walls.

—*Mohammad Elshinawy*

The story of the shifting political, architectural, and legal landscape of New York City in the wake of the attacks of September 11, 2001, will be written and rewritten.[1] Yet those who will be least visible from that narrative are the ones who bore the brunt of the backlash while also sharing the trauma of the attacks along with the rest of New Yorkers: New York City's Muslim residents.

In the immediate aftermath of September 11, the New York City Police Department (NYPD) aimed to set itself apart on the national landscape, seeking to become the leading local law enforcement agency in counterterrorism efforts, arguably competing with the federal government. A central pillar to this response was the targeting of New York City's large, diverse, and overwhelmingly immigrant Muslim American population for surveillance. Thanks to documents that have been leaked to the public, we can now read about the details of an elaborate, secret surveillance program that mapped, monitored, and analyzed American Muslim daily life throughout New York City, and surrounding areas. The intimacy of this surveillance was stark: coffee shop banter, student kayaking trips, marriage ceremonies, and private conversations were featured in NYPD files. Youth activities—and Muslim students in particular—were especially targeted. Informants or undercover officers were dispatched into all of these spaces, befriending, joining in prayer, and listening in. Student group websites, listservs, and chat rooms were infiltrated.

As the city slowly distanced itself from the attacks, picked up the pieces, and began the collective healing process, a more insidious reality settled in as the new normal: a generation of New Yorkers had grown up under the watchful gaze of the police department. They had befriended informants, learned that their personal or community spaces have been infiltrated by the state, seen their Facebook posts turn up in police files. These youth are coming of age as members of a suspect community, to borrow from Paddy Hillyard's famous 1993 study of anti-Irish policies in Britain.[2] While other communities in the United States have experienced intensive targeting and scrutiny by the state including among their youth, law enforcement's covert presence in youths' daily lives, with this degree of intimacy and deception, is arguably unprecedented in American history. Indeed, while COINTELPRO notoriously targeted black activism, much of which focused on youth groups, that surveillance was not the same blanket surveillance that left no way of opting out to the Muslim American New Yorkers, save masking their Muslim identity and silencing their religious expression. The longer-term effects are yet to be fully seen, although as this chapter reveals, their stratifying and silencing impacts call for the attention of educators, policymakers, artists, and historians alike.

The details of the NYPD's surveillance program have spurred a range of criticisms: Investigative reporters and scholars have debunked the notion that such suspicionless surveillance was effective. Even the then-chief of the NYPD Intelligence Division, Lieutenant Paul Galati, admitted during sworn testimony in 2012 that in the six years of his tenure, the unit tasked with much of this surveillance—the Demographics Unit—had not yielded a single criminal lead. Legal challenges were brought in federal courts raising constitutional and other arguments against many aspects of these practices.[3] Among the responses of supporters of surveillance was that these practices were "harmless," and that only those who had something to hide should have something to fear. Yet as any observer of totalitarian regimes knows, surveillance in and of itself, without more, has a transformative effect on its target. It serves an ordering, panoptic role. And, especially when it targets Muslim students as they develop their social and political identities, it serves a stratifying role.

This chapter moves beyond the arguments—all of them important and meritorious—that focus on the ineffectiveness and the illegality of the City's surveillance practices, and toward paying attention to the harms of surveillance. In 2011, understanding the consequences of surveillance on its targets—and the need to respond to the allegation of harmlessness—spurred my colleagues at the Creating Law Enforcement Accountability & Responsibility (CLEAR) project, a clinical project based out of City University of New York (CUNY) School of Law, our students and I to undertake a series of interviews in New York City. We set out to identify the experiences of those whose daily speech, religious practice, friendships, clothing, and behavior were put under the lens of the state. In identifying interviewees as well as verifying our findings, we drew on our organization's community-based partnerships.[4] We conducted fifty-seven semistructured interviews with Muslim religious figures, students, youth, business owners, and professionals. In particular, we reached out to individuals who frequented many of the mosques, student groups, or lived in neighborhoods that had been featured in the NYPD's documents.

The result was a fifty-four-page report entitled *Mapping Muslims, NYPD Spying and Its Impact on American Muslims*.[5] The report documented, in unprecedented detail, the chilling effect that law enforcement infiltration and mapping has on religious life, association, speech, and activism, as well as the harms it has on relationships with law enforcement, and education. Our findings were published in 2013 by CLEAR and partner organizations. They showed how surveillance chilled constitutionally protected rights—curtailing religious practice, censoring speech, and stunting political organizing. We also found that surveillance severed the trust that should exist between the police department and the communities it is charged with protecting. Finally, the report documented the stigmatizing effect that government surveillance has on the targeted communities—labeling entire communities as "suspect communities."

Of our interviews, those with New York City's Muslim youth—college-age students whose entire political awakening was in a post–9/11 world—were the most jarring, and what I delve further into in this chapter. Capitalizing on our presence at a CUNY campus and our deep community ties, we were able to hear, in great detail and greater confidence, so many of these students' deepest fears and understanding of their place as New Yorkers. In the following pages, I draw heavily on the interviews and other research that we gathered as part of the *Mapping Muslims* effort, and update them with more recent developments.

Five years since the public revelations, a reflection on the impacts of the NYPD surveillance program remains timely and is unfortunately not just backward looking. Surveillance is increasingly accepted as a post–9/11 reality. Initially provisional measures have turned into a permanent form of governance. Although New York City's experience with surveillance may be more acute than other American cities, it is certainly not aberrant. The federal government, as well as other local police departments, have engaged in similar broad-based surveillance and targeting of

Muslim populations. In fact, we now know that the FBI has similarly targeted Muslim student organizations for potential informant recruitment, seeking to recruit students to be used as "human tripwires."[6] At least until 2015, undercover officers were still infiltrating student groups, despite NYPD assertions of having implemented reforms—and the shape of its current practices is not fully known.[7]

In an era of mass surveillance, privacy and First Amendment scholars have begun to develop more robust articulations of the harms of surveillance.[8] As Edward Snowden's leaks revealing government mass surveillance, and technologically enabled tracking of activities on a massive scale has become possible, the average American has been thinking more consciously about questions of privacy and what level of government access to that data they might be comfortable with. However, the relevant experience in these inquiries tends to focus on those who are not the primary targets of surveillance: the unintended consequences of mass surveillance, how innocent passersby may be swept up in efforts to catch the targets that are assumed to be legitimate. The concerns have also articulated themselves as a (largely law-oriented) debate around the degree to which government access to metadata or location services are truly violative of privacy. Judge Richard Posner wrote that "machine collection of data cannot, as such, invade privacy."[9] However one might feel about the relative validity of that statement, a machine collection is at least very different from the private betrayal of a friend. As surveillance scholar Hewitt put it, "impersonal technological surveillance simply doesn't inspire the same pain."[10]

Muslim New Yorkers' experiences show that there is a qualitative and quantitative difference between mass surveillance and the experience of those who are intimately, deliberately, and directly targeted for surveillance. This chapter draws on our interviews, in particular those with young New Yorkers who came of age under surveillance, and details the ways in which their lives and experiences differ significantly from that of their peers.

## Background on the NYPD's Surveillance Practices

In 2001, the NYPD established a secret section within its Intelligence Division (later renamed "Intelligence Bureau"), tasked with mapping and spying on the residential, social, and business landscape of American Muslims.[11] The unit, called the Demographics Unit—which was subsequently renamed "Zone Assessment Unit"—focused explicitly on twenty-eight

listed "ancestries of interest," all populations from Muslim-majority countries, along with "American Black Muslims." The details of the program
were revealed in August 2011, through a series of news reports by the
Associated Press based on a trove of leaked NYPD documents. While the
reports were surprising in their detail and depth, the fact of surveillance
was not a surprise to those who had been its targets. Some degree of
covert surveillance had been known—whether it was through the public
revelations of some informants' identities, or frequently encountered suspicious behavior. Overt surveillance has also been a regular part of Muslim American life, particularly since the attacks of September 11, 2001:
Individuals are regularly approached by local or federal law enforcement
for questioning, such as questioning at borders, by immigration officials.
A range of federal programs that disproportionately and overwhelmingly
affect American Muslims also work as a way to track or question them.
These include overbroad terrorism databases that can affect immigration
or travel.

The NYPD, however, implemented an acute, local, and intimate version of these national surveillance programs. It sent undercover officers,
who were allegedly called "rakers," into identified neighborhoods to identify what the documents described as "hot spots": restaurants, cafes, Muslim student associations, halal shops, and hookah bars. The NYPD boasted
that it was able to recruit a force from diverse backgrounds, thus sending
police officers who could blend in to the communities they watched.[12]

The department launched various "initiatives," named after the targeted group: the "Moroccan initiative" mapped businesses that were assumed to be Moroccan, many of which were in Astoria, Queens. The
"Egyptian initiative" did the same with Egyptian businesses and went as
far as New Jersey. Officers were instructed to "listen to neighborhood
gossip" and get an overall "feel for the community." They were instructed
to visit schools and interact with business owners and patrons to "gauge
sentiment."[13]

Looking through the documents, it is clear that the common thread
across all targets is their Muslim identity. In fact, in the "Syrian Locations
of Concern" report, the document was clear that the effort excluded
the sizable Syrian Jewish population and focused on the "smaller Muslim community."[14] This targeting of the Muslim faith was based on a
theory of Muslim "radicalization" that the NYPD championed and that
has similar purchase at the federal level, despite having been shown to be
deeply flawed.[15] The radicalization theory purports to identify a trajectory
through which an individual becomes a terrorist. According to this theory,

the NYPD would take special interest in signs of Muslim religiosity, including individuals who self-identified as "salafi," student groups who
hosted certain types of speakers, and noted religious behavior. NYPD
agents documented how many times a day Muslim students prayed during
a university whitewater rafting trip, which Egyptian businesses shut their
doors for daily prayers, which restaurants played Al-Jazeera, and which
Newark businesses sold halal products and alcohol.

Muslims were only the latest targets of a long history of NYPD surveillance: Race and dissent-based surveillance has a long lineage in the
NYPD. Police surveillance of dissident and minority groups can be traced
as far back as the NYPD's "Italian Squad," founded in 1904 to monitor
the practices and activities of the city's Italian immigrants. The NYPD
also had an "anarchist squad," which focused on anarchists and labor activists. The NYPD's surveillance of political activists of various kinds—
communists, anarchists, labor activists, and civil rights activists—continued through the 1930s and the 1960s, and included the Bureau of Special
Services (BOSS). BOSS notoriously focused its investigations on dissident
groups and individuals, including the NAACP, the American Civil Liberties Union, the Fifth Avenue Peace Parade Committee, and the Lower
East Side Mobilization for Peace Action, compiling detailed profiles of
organizations and individuals. Yet the NYPD's Demographics Unit represents the most prominent instance of targeting of an entire religious
group for special monitoring.

## The NYPD's Special Focus on College Campuses

The NYPD Intelligence Division identified thirty-one Muslim Student
Associations (MSA) in the New York area, and its officers zeroed in on
seven that it listed as "of concern": Baruch College, Hunter College, La
Guardia Community College, City College, Brooklyn College, St. John's
University, and Queens College. Significantly, all but one (St. John's University) of these were part of the City University of New York (CUNY)
system, public schools that draw from New York's lower-income communities. Students at these campuses are often the first in their families to
attend college and come from working-class or immigrant backgrounds.
Among the student populations of New York's schools, they represent the
least politically connected and privileged. But they are also the schools
that recruit most locally, educating generations of New Yorkers.

The leaked NYPD documents suggest that these particular MSAs were
targeted for a range of reasons, including their choice of speakers, their

having organized "militant paintball trips," or because of a determination that their students were "politically active" or trying to revive an MSA that had gone dormant.[16] Yahoo student groups, email listservs, and blogs were monitored "as a daily routine."[17] The documents noted which speakers the students were hosting for an event, the speakers' backgrounds, political beliefs, and even the names of students who posted events online.[18]

More troublingly, the Intelligence Division sent undercover police officers and informants into MSAs and other youth groups. At City College, the NYPD dispatched an undercover to attend a whitewater rafting trip to upstate New York with students. In the notes from that trip, he reported that the students prayed at least four times a day.[19] At Brooklyn College, an undercover officer who went by "Mel" befriended the young women who were active members of the Muslim Students Association, attending their wedding parties and study groups.[20] Another informant was paid to befriend a group of Muslim students and their friends who had started a charity.[21]

Our interviews also confirmed what we learned through the press: The NYPD regularly sought to recruit students to become informants. One college student recalled a visit he received from two NYPD detectives shortly after he and his family had emigrated from Malaysia. The detectives wanted him to surf the Internet and monitor certain websites. He recalled the odd questions they put to him: "What do you think of the Shi'a? Do you think they are real Muslims? What would you do if a white American girl came to you and asked for intercourse?" After he repeatedly refused to meet with them, they eventually left him alone—until several months later, when he enrolled at a CUNY school:

> This time, they offered me 400 or 500 dollars a month, they said "all your work would require would be sitting in front of your computer and look at what people are doing." . . . Within four meetings I moved from being a suspect to someone they wanted to pay.—Jamal*, 23, CUNY student

Another young woman we interviewed recounted how when she was sixteen, she got a call from the principal's office at her public school. The principal told her that the NYPD had asked her to come in for questioning. She had assumed that it was in response to her complaints about someone who had been stalking her. However, once there, she found that the officers were more interested in her and her friends' online activities. A few weeks later, the same NYPD officers that she spoke to at her school came to her home while her parents were away. They searched through her belongings and her computer and ultimately offered her work as an informant. She described how at the time, this was a very enticing offer, in particular as she was poor and living with her parents:

> [The detective] said the department can provide you with a place, a job if that's what you're looking for, an apartment, we can give you your freedom.—Grace★, 23, Queens resident

Grace then articulated a sentiment that was common across MSA students—even though they had not yet obtained the leaked internal NYPD documents, or known the extent of the programs. They and their peers' experiences made it seem inevitable that they were constantly surrounded by informants:

> Everyone is being asked to spy, and I know it myself they must have been threatened or bribed to spy. Nobody would just do it voluntarily. And they probably get people in trouble. I know this because they tried to bribe me.—Grace★, 23, Queens resident

Finally, recent leaked documents show that it was not just the NYPD but also the federal government that have identified college students as ideal informants.[22] Thus, students—who already faced surveillance in their neighborhoods, in their home setting, and in their mosques—were also experiencing this surveillance perhaps most intensively on their campuses.

## Chilling Religious Practice and Study

> An informer system is not only a means of collecting information, but its most effective social function perhaps is the general fear it produces.[23]

We found, perhaps unsurprisingly, that surveillance of Muslims' quotidian activities has created a pervasive climate of fear and suspicion, in particular on college campuses.

Perhaps the most obvious area of impact was the impact of surveillance on students' religious life and expression. The NYPD's spotlight on how individuals practiced their faith, their degree of religiosity and their places of worship disrupted Muslims' ability to practice freely. Interviewees, no matter how young, showed an acute awareness of the direct badge of suspicion accorded to religious practice:

> It's as if the law says: the more Muslim you are, the more trouble you can be, so decrease your Islam.—Sari★, 19, Brooklyn College

I can't grow my beard, I'll get in trouble. I can't dress like this, I can't talk like that ... It's stressful.—Kaled Refat, 24, New Jersey resident

When I was on the MSA board, we were two niqabis [women who wear the face veil] and two brothers with big beards. I've heard from some people that they thought we were *salafi*—but that's just because we looked the part. Technically, we weren't. But that's how we were labeled and I think that's how the NYPD has labeled us, too.—Asma*, 19, CUNY student

Within heterogeneous Muslim communities, this resulted in the suppression of certain practices of Islam more than others, with the more conservative individuals bearing the brunt of the burden. Younger interviewees described how parents warned them about appearing "too Muslim" or forbade them from attending Muslim student group events or wearing traditional Muslim clothing. One Queens College student who wears the *niqab*, or face veil, noted that her mother asked her to stop wearing all black because she worried her dress would make her a target for surveillance, whereas her mother was not as concerned about her brother because "he doesn't necessarily 'look Muslim.'"

Many students we interviewed also discussed fear of discussing important religious concepts. For example, the word *jihad*, a central concept in Islam, translates from Arabic as "to strive" or "to struggle." The term is used as a term denoting an effort, endeavor, or struggle to improve one's own religious practice. Yet it has prominently been reduced, often by the press and in other public debates, to only refer to a violent struggle. It is a concept and term that calls for debate, explanation, and elaboration. The negative attention brought to the term has placed it at the center of law enforcement interest. As a result, many students we interviewed described avoiding using the term altogether. This means that they avoid exploring, expanding, and debating a key religious concept.

We don't use the word jihad. Sometimes speakers will steer away from that word, or make extra effort to explain it more, explain exactly what we mean, so that nobody can misinterpret or get the wrong idea, especially in larger gatherings.—Amira,* 22, Sunday school teacher

I don't talk about the concept of jihad. But anytime someone asks that question, my first reaction is to deflect that question to someone else who can answer without me having to talk about it. Because of the known things that happen when you talk about jihad, it's one of those words that can trigger automatic surveillance.— Jawad Rasul, 25, CUNY student

## Impact on Campus Life

Another key finding was how surveillance has a chilling effect on freedom of speech and expression on campuses. Our interviews showed that college students became afraid to discuss matters that were deemed overtly political, including civil rights issues or international affairs. Surveillance has interfered in how and whether they make the meaningful friendships that are typically developed in college and that might last a lifetime. Professors described this chilling of student life as "devastating" to the student experience in and out of the classroom. College, for most, is when students begin to experiment with their political identities, their beliefs, self-expression, and opinions. They test out their voices, and they become involved in causes that may result in fundamental shifts in their life and career choices. They learn how to lead, how to navigate institutions, and how to be citizens. The post–9/11 climate of surveillance and close scrutiny has deterred scores of American Muslims from developing their leadership skills and mobilizing for social causes. The long-term effects of these phenomena on these students and their communities have yet to be fully seen or understood.

It is perhaps the sense of community and belonging that is the first casualty during what is an already fraught college experience. This is particularly the case for those exploring new identities, including those who converted to Islam during college.

> I was very naive at one point. I converted to Islam. At first I thought all Muslims were great people and you could trust them all. And then someone said hey, you should know about all these things (referring to informants) . . . —Hassan★, 20, board member of a CUNY MSA

Two interviewees recalled incidents where they falsely accused someone of being an informant, leading to potentially devastating reputational consequences for the accused. One of the students, who was on a whitewater rafting trip, was asked during a press interview on national television that followed the revelation of the NYPD's infiltration of his trip whether he knew who the undercover was. He ventured a guess, and he was wrong. When speaking with us, he expressed remorse: "I have to give him a call and apologize."[24]

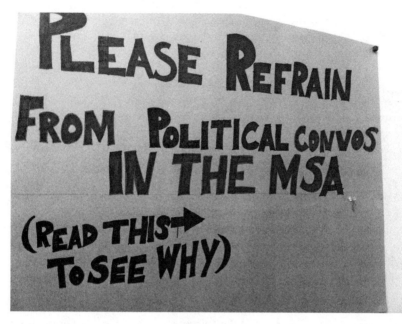

Figure 1. Sign in the Muslim Students Association (MSA) Room at Hunter College, New York City. "Read this" pointed to a printout of a press article about the NYPD surveillance program. Credit: Fouzia Najar

## Chilled Student Activism

Interviewees noted self-censorship of political speech and activism. The stifling and self-censorship of both routine and political speech have especially dire consequences for college students as political activism, student organizing and academic pursuits are derailed during the most formative years of a young person's life. Students have found themselves unable to organize effectively or even to respond to news of surveillance, often times directly linking their silencing to the knowledge of NYPD surveillance (Figure 1).

> The [NYPD's] MSA documents say we are becoming more political, we want to avoid that.—Jamal★, 23, CUNY student

> At the Muslim Student Organization it's a given that you don't touch a sensitive topic.—Jawad Rasul, 25, CUNY student

> We don't bring up politics aside from humanitarian causes like natural disasters, and then we just remind others to pray for others. —Samia★, 21, CUNY student[25]

Interviewees noted steering clear from conversations relating to foreign policy, civil rights and activism, and even surveillance. This same fear deterred mobilization around Muslim civil-rights issues on campus and quelled demands for police accountability. Surveillance, in this way, ensured more surveillance as it created a space void of calls for accountability.

This was particularly stark among the younger interviewees: Many noted that their parents discouraged them from being active in Muslim student groups, protests, or other activism, including being outspoken on political issues affecting Muslims in America, believing that these activities would threaten to expose them to government scrutiny. Such fears were heightened among parents who came from immigrant backgrounds, fearing that their children's outspokenness on political matters or surveillance might be unsafe or might trigger immigration consequences.

> At [the] Youth Center, a girl said that the idea of being arrested isn't something that's far fetched, that's unbelievable; it's something very real, very possible for her. She thought it was really important to lay low because it would break her mom's heart if she got arrested. . . . "Laying low" means not being politically active, literally going on with their everyday lives. A lot of people feel like being at these protests is counterproductive, that it would draw more attention, more of being spied on.—Sireen★, 23, student at Hunter College[26]

This silencing effect is exacerbated by the vulnerability or lack of privilege that students on CUNY campuses feel. They couldn't rely on connected parents or well-resourced schools to protect them. As one longtime CUNY faculty member told us:

> CUNY students are so grateful to be in CUNY in the first place. They don't want to rock the boat. The last thing they want to do is anything that would endanger their chances of getting an education.[27]

Faculty and student government bodies were vociferous in their condemnation of the news of spying. They made several calls on the CUNY system to provide better protection to its students and demanded guarantees of nonrepetition.[28] Such university involvement continues to this day, Brooklyn College's student-run paper still regularly reporting on the fallout of the NYPD's surveillance program.[29] However, only the NYPD could ultimately provide that certainty.

In addition to muting themselves on campus, students reported withdrawing from engaging with their non-Muslim classmates and colleagues. One of the major components of the mission of any Muslim Student Association is to engage non-Muslims on their campus and to increase the Muslim community's visibility.[30] Students worried that wide press coverage announcing that the NYPD had infiltrated Muslim student groups with the hope of finding radicals or criminals would damage their outreach efforts. Several interviewees noted feeling that many on campus did not want to associate with the MSA or its active members.[31]

For college students, typically aged between seventeen and twenty-two, the prospect of dealing with surveillance by a police department, infiltration of events and extracurricular activities by informants, and the potentially devastating academic, professional, and personal repercussions can be overwhelming. This section discusses some of the ways in which Muslim students' lives have been affected on campuses and how Muslim students' college experience—and education—is significantly different from their non-Muslim peers' as a result of NYPD surveillance. We found that the NYPD's surveillance of students chilled First Amendment activity in what is perhaps the single most important formative and expressive space for any American youth: the college campus.

## Responding to the News

With the first round of press reports unveiling the NYPD's infiltration of seven MSAs in the City University of New York (CUNY) system, MSA leaders were hesitant to speak out.[32] Tensions were high on the various campuses, as the college students deliberated how to respond to the national headlines publicizing that the NYPD considers them to be potentially dangerous. Although many members of CUNY faculties and student governments spoke out in solidarity with the Muslim student groups, the official administrations were less quick to condemn covert NYPD activities on their campuses. MSA leaders we spoke with described being torn about how to respond under such circumstances.

> On the one hand you don't want people to be afraid, while on the other hand you don't want them to be too naïve.—Soheeb Amin, 22, former President of a CUNY MSA

Some MSAs limited their response to inviting local attorneys and civil rights organizations such as CLEAR to facilitate "Know Your Rights" workshops. Yet even holding these events was sometimes controversial. On one campus, a student leader told us that his group opted to not record these events despite their normal policy of doing so, in order to protect the students. Several students noted a general hesitation to address surveillance on their campus. Interviewees also noted that, as a matter of policy, many MSA boards refrained from hosting "political" conversations and events. They reasoned that where their group was already under surveillance, such conversations would be recorded and misconstrued, and, if their group was not under surveillance, political conversations by a Muslim group would trigger surveillance or have the group identified as "extremist." Student groups were cognizant of the unwarranted attention controversial discussions might attract from peers.

## Chilled Academic Expression

Our research found, perhaps unsurprisingly, that surveillance of Muslims' political opinions had devastating effects on classroom dynamics, and stunted students' personal and academic growth. Discussions, debates, exchanges, political and theoretical experimentation, and even role-playing and posturing are critical aspects of a healthy educational environment. Several of the students we interviewed described self-censoring classroom comments not only because of a fear of law enforcement scrutiny. Yet others noted a concern that other classmates or professors would misinterpret their views, given the ambient discourse on young, overtly political Muslims.[33]

One college student noted that she would check with her friend who worked at a Muslim civil-rights organization ahead of submitting her papers for school, or even ahead of choosing her paper topics. She was advised to write freely, while also keeping in mind that her papers might be shared with the police department. One of the students who was on the whitewater rafting trip that was infiltrated by an NYPD undercover told us:

> Colleges are a place where these discussions are supposed to happen so people can learn from each other. We're losing out.—Jawad Rasul, 25, CUNY student

Similar observations played out for how student groups chose their speakers and their events. For example, they refrained from inviting speakers that would be deemed to be "salafi" to their campus events. Such a concern was not unfounded: in its policy paper "Radicalization in the West," the NYPD explicitly identified certain routine American Muslim behaviors as suspicious and broadly characterized these behaviors as Salafi.[34] The NYPD then claimed that anyone who participates in these Salafi behaviors might be exhibiting indicators of "radicalization." The conflation between religious ideology, religious practice, and indicators of potential criminal activity was not lost on the students we spoke with:

> We try to position ourselves by thinking whether the NYPD is going to think the speaker is Salafi, or whether the person has training from Saudi, that might give us unwanted attention from the NYPD.
> —Jamal*, 23, CUNY student

Two students we spoke with, both active members of their MSAs, reported switching their majors from political science to more conventional majors after becoming concerned about law enforcement scrutiny of "political" young Muslim males.

Jeanne Theoharis noticed a retreat from nonprofessional degrees, even as secondary concentrations, among her Muslim students at Brooklyn College. In largely immigrant communities where social and familial pressures are to direct oneself toward professional degrees—business administration, accounting, engineering, or medicine—a secondary concentration or extracurricular activities have always been a way for students to explore their passions or their interests in other directions.

These impacts aren't limited to the Muslim students. Their peers, their teachers, and the intellectual community as a whole suffer when diverse views are stifled. Professors noted that students are concerned about speaking in class, or general reticence or anxiety around certain discussions, in particular those deemed "political."

> Israel/Palestine and Muslim youth culture are the two topics where you feel the air goes out of the room. Students get anxious. The conversation is uncomfortable, the atmosphere changes in the room.
> —Carla Bellamy, Professor, Baruch College

## Poisoned College Experiences

MSA offices and prayer rooms are intended to be safe spaces for Muslim students to come together, support each other and talk freely about issues affecting their community. This need is especially important on CUNY campuses with large student bodies spread out over urban campuses, or where the resources devoted to extracurricular activities might be slimmer. Infiltration of MSAs by undercover police officers and informants is a blow to the groups' core function. On some campuses, interviewees noted drops in attendance at MSA events in the immediate aftermath of the Associated Press reports.[35]

[The upperclassmen] told us we encourage you to have free speech and political conversations, just not inside the MSA room. Because we don't want an informant to be here to catch one of your lines or crazy rants and you would get in trouble. I don't want to go to the MSA room because I'm worried that someone will report what I'm saying. . . . The MSA felt more awkward for everyone. No one was talking about it but we knew there was a problem, we were just scared to say something.—Fatima★, 19, CUNY student

At Brooklyn College, the college paper reported that following the Associated Press stories about on-campus surveillance, the annual "Islam Awareness Week" events were significantly less well attended than previous years, and that speakers requested not to be identified by name or have their photographs taken.[36]

Though the feelings of suspicion toward others are corrosive to any community, students' youth and the fragility of their nascent social ties make it particularly destructive in the college setting. College is a place where students typically forge lifelong friendships and explore social, religious and political identities and groups. Students we spoke with were ever cognizant that an undercover officer or informant might be among them. Several students noted that either a sudden surge or a sudden drop in someone's MSA activity would make them suspicious of that person.

It made me feel hostile to other MSA members. I didn't know who to trust anymore. —Fatima★, 19, CUNY student

Our students are convinced that there must be spies or undercover agents. . . . We have a huge student body, it's impossible to know everyone. They also note that many students have financial concerns, and are thus likely to be pressured to become informants.—Jamal★, 23, CUNY student

Because of this atmosphere, students observed that their MSA is not able to fulfill its role as a support group or as a safe space to discuss the very issues that are silencing them. One interviewee was a young man who had the NYPD come to his home to question him about his political opinions and who had, as a result, withdrawn from all public events. He described the atmosphere when he finally mustered the courage to attend an MSA event after a long absence. He said that "people were looking at [him] funny because they hadn't seen [him] before" and may have thought he was an informant.

The suspicion and mistrust that surveillance breeds also stifled opportunities for reaching out across student groups and communities, including for support:

> Even to bring all the MSAs in one room, we're not going to trust them. From one MSA to another, you'll need to establish trust. Where do you start doing that? A CUNY-wide Know-Your-Rights event would be great, but because of the lack of trust anything more than that would be difficult. We would be wondering who is writing what down, what meaning would be imposed on the words, who would come and knock on their doors next.—Samia*, 21, CUNY student

> I don't want to be sitting at a roundtable, I'll just be wondering whether someone will be secretly taking notes and sending it God knows where. They would write "that girl thinks this."—then whose door are they going to knock on? —Inas*, 20, CUNY student

## The Intimacy of Betrayal via Informant

As students learned that their classmates or friends had been undercover officers or informants, an atmosphere of mistrust settled in. What was striking in our discussions with Muslim students was the intimacy of the betrayal they experienced. The force of betrayal is significantly more powerful than other forms of monitoring, no matter how intrusive they might be. Hewitt has argued that it is precisely that destructive, divisive, and non-neutral nature of informants that makes them such an appealing counterterrorism tool.[37] On campuses, the intensity of the friendship bonds and relationships made this aspect all the more devastating.

One nineteen-year-old student who was caught on a marijuana possession charge was "turned" into an informant and infiltrated a number of different college-age circles around New York City. Eventually, he "outed" himself on Facebook, shocking many of the students whom he had befriended and on whom he was spying. One of the students he befriended, who eventually became a plaintiff in a lawsuit against the NYPD, told us:

> I met him (the informant) through the MSA's Facebook connections. He had told me he wanted to become a better person and to strengthen his faith. So I took him in, introduced him to all of my friends, got him involved in our extracurricular activities. I would

wake him up for prayer every morning. He even slept over at my house, and I let him in even though he smelled of marijuana but I tried to look past it because I knew he was new to Islam. When I was texted the news (that he was an informant), the shock caused me to drop my phone. It took me 24 hours to get myself together and to respond, everyone on Facebook was waiting to hear what I would say, because I'm the one who introduced him to them.—Asad Dandia, 19, CUNY student[38]

Perhaps the most striking illustration of the intimacy of this betrayal occurred after our research and report were concluded. In 2016, a group of young alumnae at Brooklyn College learned that their friend and confidante from their college years was actually an NYPD undercover officer all along. The undercover agent, a woman who went by the name of "Mel," posed as a recent convert to Islam with Turkish origins. She befriended them, attended bridal showers, visited their homes, and became an integral part of their college experience. This information was not obtained through leaked documents—rather, her identity was revealed after the students recognized her in press reports about a prosecution of two young women on terrorism related charges. The NYPD has confirmed that they had deployed an informant to infiltrate Brooklyn College's Muslim student group for a year, not yielding any investigations.[39]

And yet, as we were interviewing Brooklyn College students, some of the very same women who had befriended her had spoken with my colleagues and me about their concerns about informants, even describing, in vague and secretive terms, this specific young woman. As we listened to them, the students were struggling to balance their concerns about a woman they described as having odd behavior and asking intrusive and invasive questions, with their desire to abide by what they believe to be their faith-based obligation to not engage in gossip. Years later, as these young women's suspicions turned out to be true, they have bravely and publicly spoken up about their ordeals. In recalling Mel's behavior with the benefit of hindsight, the women have been able to piece together a much clearer picture. Jeanne Theoharis, a professor at Brooklyn College who became an important resource for her students as they were responding to the deeply personal and communal harm of these developments, wrote:

Mel wormed her way into their friendships, their trips to Coney Island, their picnics and jokes. She even became a bridesmaid in one woman's wedding. She inquired about their politics and mimicked their religious practices. Claiming she'd been raised in a secular Muslim Turkish family but now wanted to embrace Islam, she recited the Shahada, a declaration of Muslim faith, at the first meeting many students remember her attending, and later spent dozens of hours "praying" next to them. She participated in clubs on campus, joined numerous listservs, and invited students to go with her to events around the city.[40]

The story of these young women at Brooklyn College has been well documented thanks to an unlikely alignment of facts with the official "outing" of Mel, a group of brave and outspoken students, support from engaged faculty, and thoughtful journalists and documentarians who also sought to tell their story.[41] However, it is unfortunately not unique. Those we interviewed had almost unanimously observed an atmosphere where everyone scrutinizes everyone, directing particular hesitation and suspicion toward new faces in the community, converts to Islam, or anyone perceived to be an outsider. Many interviewees admitted to shunning individuals who behaved differently, perhaps even awkwardly. Someone who expressed particular interest in political topics or curiosity about their Islamic faith became a cause for concern, rather than embraced. Similarly, some described an aversion to those who appeared overtly religious or political because they were assumed to be more likely targets of surveillance.

## The Stratifying, Stigmatizing Role of Surveillance

They say "don't you go to Queens College? Isn't that where all the terrorists are?" They saw it on the news that they were spying on us.

If they [weren't] already monitoring me, now that I'm in the MSA at Queens College, I'm definitely monitored.—Sameera*, 19, CUNY student

Debates about the merits of surveillance put a primacy on the loss of privacy—and that is certainly a concern here, especially to the student who suddenly finds out that what she thought were her private conversations with a friend were actually being recorded. Such privacy harms are primarily experienced at the individual, interpersonal level. However, the state's betrayal also presents communal harms. Among them is how it entrenches social stratification. David Lyon has called this social sorting, a "key means of reproducing and reinforcing social, economic, and cultural divisions in informational societies."[42] Indeed, when focused on marginalized communities, surveillance does not ignite controversy—except within those targeted communities where surveillance and informants can be divisive and destructive. If the state were to expand the targets of its surveillance, its efforts will likely not pass muster. This was arguably what happened with the short-lived Terrorism Information and Prevention System (TIPS) program, a George W. Bush–era program that aimed to enlist various professions to report information encountered over the course of their jobs to the government. American lawmakers and critics characterized this as an effort to enlist Americans to "spy on one another."[43] That program was ultimately canceled.

Some have posited that the difference between the surveillance practices of a liberal democracy and those of a totalitarian regime is not so much in the techniques used, but in the scope of their reach and who they target.[44] A totalitarian regime subjects its entire population to surveillance, whereas in a liberal democracy, invasive techniques are limited to politically marginalized groups. Policy decisions around matters relating to counterterrorism surveillance are often discussed as striking a balance between security and privacy, or security and liberty. "On the one hand, it is creepy, Orwellian, and corrosive of civil liberties. On the other hand, it keeps us and our children safe."[45] The problem with this fallacy is that groups that are usually not involved in decision making around what balance to strike disproportionately shoulder the costs. In other words, it is an easier cost to accept if it is not one that is being directly experienced. The other problem with this framing is the assumption that surveillance yields safety, when it has not been shown to do so—certainly not in the context of the NYPD's surveillance program.

There is also something about the spying being at the hands of a local police department as opposed to the federal government that increases the stratifying effects of surveillance. The NYPD is tasked with protecting New Yorkers. By associating itself with deception and covert activity, some of the most vulnerable segments of New York's immigrant communities are essentially deprived of the protections of their local police department. Variants of this argument have been recognized in the context of immigration enforcement, as immigrant-rights advocates and police departments alike have recognized the harms of enlisting local police departments to do the work of federal immigration enforcement agencies. In that context, many local police departments (including the NYPD) have declined participating in immigration enforcement. A similar analysis has yet to be developed in the context of the NYPD's surveillance program.

However, the unique harms that flow from police surveillance were certainly identified by the young people we interviewed:

> Now that it's the NYPD it's a lot closer to home. It's more local. You don't know how to differentiate between the two. . . . Usually, police officers, you ask them for directions, they're around on campus. Now, how am I supposed to differentiate between the NYPD and the FBI? People don't understand how different it is that a local law enforcement agency is doing this.—Fareeda*, 21, Brooklyn College student

## Conclusion

In March 2017, after years of community organizing and accompanying litigation, the NYPD reached a settlement in two lawsuits challenging the legality of its surveillance program. The terms of the settlement established a number of reforms to the police department's rules that aim to limit the police department's ability to engage in suspicionless surveillance, and increase oversight of the NYPD's intelligence division. While these are important changes, the longer-term impacts of NYPD surveillance, in particular of Muslim students, are yet to be fully seen. A generation of American Muslim youth has adjusted how they go about their studies, partake in extracurricular activities, choose their professions, engage with their classmates, and develop their social roles and relationships. Our report observed that the isolationism that comes with being a member of a "spied on" community means that Muslim students are getting a fundamentally different and less rewarding college experience compared to their non-Muslim peers. That has long term and immeasurable impacts on the city's social fabric and institutions. These impacts remain understudied.

### Notes

This article draws on research that I conducted with colleagues and students while I worked at the Creating Law Enforcement Accountability & Responsibility (CLEAR) project at the CUNY School of Law. Our research culminated in a 2013 report, *Mapping Muslims: NYPD Spying and Its Impact on American Muslims.* Nermeen Arastu and I coauthored that report, with editorial support from Amna Akbar and Ramzi Kassem.

1. The quotation from Mohammad Elshinawy is taken from in-court testimony delivered on April 19, 2016, speaking in support of a joint settlement reached in two separate lawsuits: *Raza et al. v. City of New York et al.*, No. 13-

cv-3448 (March 20, 2017, E.D.N.Y.), and *Handschu v. Special Services Division*, 71-cv-2203 (March 13, 2017, S.D.N.Y.).

2. Hillyard, 1993.

3. *Raza v. City of New York*; *Handschu v. Special Services Division*; *Hassan v. City of New York* (Third Circuit, Oct. 13, 2015). The author and my colleagues at CLEAR were counsel for plaintiffs in *Raza v. City of New York*.

4. All interviewees were given the option of being interviewed anonymously. The overwhelming majority of our interviewees opted for anonymity, some on the further condition that we not disclose even generic information about them, including their class year, college, or country of origin. This request was as common for young students with foreign-born parents as it was for well-established and affluent young professionals, and even civil rights attorneys. To honor these concerns, we used aliases for those interviewees who requested to remain anonymous. In addition, we have scrubbed details that might identify a particular mosque or Muslim students' association to respect the privacy of other members whom we have not necessarily interviewed but whose interests are implicated in the representation of their community or sentiments.

5. Shamas and Arastu, 2013.

6. Federal Bureau of Investigations, n.d. *See also* Cora Currier, "The FBI Wanted to Target Yemenis through Student Groups and Mosques," *The Intercept*, September 29, 2016.

7. Aviva Stahl, "NYPD Undercover 'Converted' to Islam to Spy on Brooklyn College Students," *The Gothamist,* October 29, 2015.

8. *See, e.g.,* Richards, 2013; Solove, 2008.

9. Richard Posner, "Our Domestic Intelligence Crisis," *Washington Post,* December 21, 2005.

10. Hewitt, 2010, 120.

11. Many of the documents that were leaked to the press are available on the Associated Press website, as part of a series of Pulitzer Prize-winning reporting: https://goo.gl/LaAh2L.

12. *Handschu v. Special Services Division*, Deposition of Galati, 68–69.

13. Shamas and Arastu, 2013, 10.

14. New York Police Department Intelligence Division, Syrian Locations of Concern, https://goo.gl/EqkzsX.

15. Silber and Bhatt, n.d.

16. Shamas and Arastu, 2013, 40.

17. New York City Police Department, Weekly MSA Report (2006).

18. Ibid.

19. Chris Hawley, "NYPD Monitored Muslim Students All over Northeast," *Associated Press*, February 18, 2012.

20. Jeanne Theoharis, "'I Feel like a Despised Insect': Coming of Age under Surveillance in New York," *The Intercept,* February 18, 2016.

21. Asad Dandia, "My Life Under NYPD Surveillance: A Brooklyn Student and Charity Leader on Fear and Mistrust," *American Civil Liberties Union,* June 18, 2013.

22. Currier, "FBI Wanted to Target Yemenis."

23. Akerstrom, 1991.

24. Shamas and Arastu, 2013, 26.

25. Ibid., 41.

26. Ibid., 23.

27. Ibid., 42.

28. Zainab Iqbal, "Two Years Later, Brooklyn College Looks Back on NYPD's Surveillance of Muslims," *The Excelsior,* November 8, 2017.

29. Ahmed Aly, "Professors Explain Surveillance on Campus and First Amendment Rights," *The Kingsman,* February 28, 2017.

30. Shamas and Arastu, 2013, 43.

31. Ibid., 44–45.

32. Ibid., 41–42.

33. Ibid., 44–45.

34. Silber and Bhatt, n.d.

35. Shamas and Arastu, 2013, 42.

36. Ibid.

37. Hewitt, 2010, 124.

38. Shamas and Arastu, 2013, 40.

39. Aviva Stahl, "Brooklyn College Students: NYPD Illegally Spied on Us & Lied about It," *The Gothamist,* January 5, 2016.

40. Jeanne Theoharis, "I Feel like a Despised Insect."

41. Mitchell and Varga, n.d.

42. Hewitt, 2010, 136.

43. Nat Hentoff, "*The Death of Operation TIPS,*" *Village Voice,* December 17, 2002.

44. Hewitt, 2010, 120.

45. Richards, 2013.

## References

Akerstrom, Malin. *Betrayal and Betrayers: The Sociology of Treachery.* London: Transaction Publishers, 1991.

Federal Bureau of Investigation. "Responding to the Yemeni Threat, Scenarios for CHS Development." https://goo.gl/dDziLj.

Hewitt, Steve. *Snitch! A History of the Modern Intelligence Informer.* New York: Continuum, 2010.

Hillyard, Paddy. *Suspect Community: People's Experience of the Prevention of Terrorism Acts in Britain.* London: Pluto Press, 1993.

Mitchell, Katie, and Danielle Varga. *Watched, Coming of Age, under the Gaze of State Surveillance: The Documentary.* https://goo.gl/rU15dh.

Richards, Neil. "The Dangers of Surveillance." *Harvard Law Review* 126 (2013): 1934–1965.

Shamas, Diala, and Nermeen Arastu. *Mapping Muslims: NYPD Spying and Its Impact on American Muslims.* New York: CLEAR, MACLC, AALDEF, 2013. Available at https://goo.gl/jxyXcy.

Silber, Mitchell, and Arvind Bhatt. *Radicalization in the West: The Homegrown Threat.* New York: New York Police Department, n.d.

Solove, Daniel. "Data Mining and the Security-Liberty Debate." *University of Chicago Law Review* 75 (2008): 343–362.

# Memory, Site, and Object
## The September 11 Memorial Museum

Susan Opotow and Karyna Pryiomka

The September 11 Memorial Museum is situated in Lower Manhattan at the site where the World Trade Center's Twin Towers stood. From 1973 to 2001 the Towers were an international economic hub symbolizing America's economic strength and political power.[1] Each was 110 stories high and together contained 10 million square feet of space that accommodated 50,000 workers and 200,000 visitors daily. On September 11, 2001, the Twin Towers were destroyed in a terrorist attack that killed close to three thousand people. Many more were sickened and died from environmental aftereffects of the buildings' collapse in the months and years that followed.[2]

The September 11 Memorial Museum opened in May 2014, twelve and a half years after the 9/11 attacks. Its mission is to bear witness to the 1993 and 2001 terrorist attacks on the World Trade Center site and to honor victims of those attacks, those who risked their lives to save others, and the thousands of survivors.[3]

The September 11 Memorial Museum has four key elements: an entry pavilion on the memorial plaza, an immense void situated below the plaza, and two exhibition spaces situated within the void.[4] The entry pavilion is a striking glass structure designed by architectural firm Snøhetta. Situated on the memorial plaza designed by Michael Arad and Peter Walker, the pavilion contains an auditorium and café and leads to 127,000 square feet of underground space designed by the architectural firm Davis Brody Bond. This space descends nearly seventy feet from the memorial plaza to the footprint of the Twin Towers at bedrock where two exhibitions, the Memorial and Historical Exhibitions, are situated.

Several teams worked on various aspects of the museum's design. Thinc, the lead exhibition designer, collaborated with Local Projects to develop digital displays for the museum exhibitions. Together, they designed the Memorial Exhibition located within the footprint of the South Tower, which features photographs and biographical information on the 2,983 victims of the attacks on the World Trade Center on February 26, 1993, and September 11, 2001.[5] Layman Design developed the museum's Historical Exhibition based on early designs by Thinc. Located in the footprint of the North Tower, the Historical Exhibition features artifacts, images, first-person testimonies, and archival recordings that recount the events of 9/11.[6] The exhibition designers worked closely with the museum's curatorial staff as these exhibitions were being developed.[7]

This chapter focuses on the development of the vast underground space, an artifact of the World Trade Center's construction in 1966, that held the Twin Towers before September 11, 2001. Now encompassing the Memorial and Historical Exhibitions and other areas, this large open space represents the history of 9/11 to people throughout the world since the museum opened in 2014.[8] Our interest in the museum's design and development emerges from our work as social psychologists interested in how museums speak to a difficult past.[9] Understanding the development of the September 11 Memorial Museum clarifies how the museum's approach to design enables visitors and the larger society to contend with its traumatic past.

To learn about the museum's development and design, we spoke with architect Mark Wagner of Davis Brody Bond, whose work on the design of the museum began in 2004. His involvement with the World Trade Tower began even earlier. In 2001 he had been working for a design firm that was as a consultant for Port Authority of New York and New Jersey, the owner of the World Trade Center site. In the days after the September 11 attack, he was tasked with identifying and tagging art and artifacts in the enormous pile of debris left after the Towers' collapse that should be preserved.[10] During the nine-month cleanup period, he therefore sought out artistic or historical material that could convey what happened on September 11 to future generations and tagged approximately two thousand artifacts, including fire trucks and bent steel beams from the Towers[11] (Figure 1).

In 2004 Mark Wagner was subsequently invited by Steven Davis and Carl Krebs, partners at Davis Brody Bond, to join the team commissioned to design the space that had been beneath the Twin Towers. Because of his knowledge of the site and its artifacts, he was tasked with the

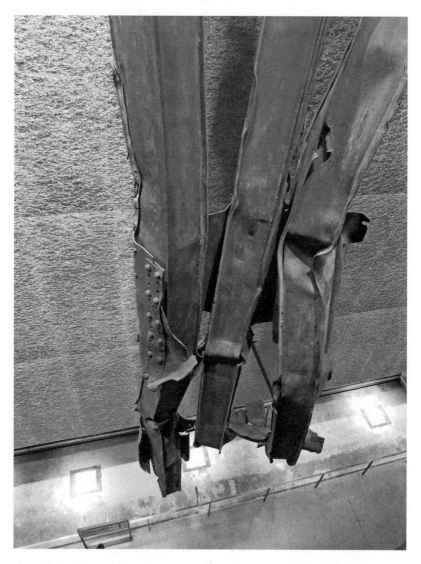

Figure 1. Steel beams from the World Trade Center site. Credit: Susan Opotow

conceptualization and program for the project, and during the construction administration phase, he led design/documentation and construction efforts. He is therefore uniquely positioned to describe the history, design, and development of the September 11 Memorial Museum in the decade from 2004 to 2014.

We met with Mark Wagner in October 2017 at Davis Brody Bond headquarters in Lower Manhattan. Through our interview with him, we describe key aspects of the museum's development, including design ideas, construction and conservation challenges, historical designations, community engagement, and environmental challenges from his insider's perspective. In the next section of the chapter we discuss how the design of the museum resonates with scholarly work on the relationship between past and present and between people and site. We conclude by describing the relevance of this scholarship to a new and prominent museum charged with representing a traumatic history to visitors.

## Goals and Challenges: Building the September 11 Memorial Museum

When Mark Wagner arrived at the site of the World Trade Towers a week and a half after the September 11 attack on the Towers, he walked past barricades on the West Side Highway where people were clustered at a perimeter fence several blocks from the World Trade Center site. Though these people did not have site access, they were there to witness what was happening. Many carried signs of support for rescue workers. As work on the site progressed, the perimeter fence was moved closer to the void until people behind the fence were standing at the site's edge and could look into the void. This image of people at the perimeter pressing to look into the void informed Mark Wagner's work on the design of the September 11 Memorial Museum.

*The Size of the Site*

From the very beginning of their work, the architects understood that the void in the ground was not just a sixteen-acre construction site in Lower Manhattan. They saw the void, the largest artifact from 9/11, as a metaphor for the enormity of loss experienced after 9/11. Because of its emotional significance, preserving the integrity of the void and its long views was a key element of the museum's design. It proved to be a key challenge as well.

When Davis Brody Bond was commissioned to design the museum in 2004, the architectural team had to act quickly to secure space for the museum. It would otherwise have been filled in with mechanical equipment, pumps, the chiller plant, and the like.[12] "It felt like a land grab," Mark Wagner said, as it was a competitive process. The question "Who needs that space more?" pitted the site's historical significance against infrastructure uses and commercial interests. As Mark Wagner describes, the architectural team "got in there and stood with our arms holding the walls back, trying to preserve open space." Securing it was the critical first step in the museum's development.

## The Ramp: Entryway to the Museum

In the aftermath of 9/11, a site access ramp was built from the south end of the site into the middle of the North Tower footprint. Initially built to provide access to the lowest level of the site for ambulances and fire trucks to take victims out, it was subsequently used by cleanup and recovery workers who walked or drove down. Mark Wagner explained that going down the ramp "you felt the emotional weight of everything was shifting as you were going from a busy city street down to some point that was very empty and quiet down below." Because of the site's solemn significance, the architects wanted visitors to experience this shift in emotional weight during their descent to bedrock. They therefore designed a slow and progressive disclosure of the museum's vast space and its contents that recreated the experience of walking down the site access ramp. Though unplanned, the museum ramp is close in length to the site access ramp, the distance, Mark Wagner observed, between the bustling city outside and the emotional experience of the museum.

## Foundation Hall, the Slurry Wall, and the Last Column

Visitors entering the museum do not see everything at once. They first see the museum's vast space from the distance. Their descent down to bedrock almost seventy feet below street level gradually reveals the size of Foundation Hall (Figure 2) and the artifacts it contains. When tons of debris were finally removed from the site, this void was all that remained. At various vantage points along the ramp, visitors can stand at the perimeter and look into Foundation Hall, with 15,000 square feet of floor space and forty- to sixty-foot-high ceilings. Its open space contains objects connected with the site, including the bedrock in which the Twin Towers

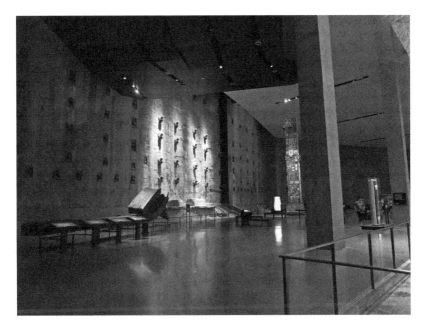

Figure 2. Foundation Hall. Credit: Susan Opotow

were anchored, the slurry wall that had prevented the Hudson River from flooding the site during construction and after, steel beams that were contorted in the 9/11 attack, and the last column removed when the site cleanup was completed in May 2002. The emptiness of this space can help visitors grasp what no longer exists and the enormity of that destruction.

After 9/11, the site had contained tons of debris from the building's catastrophic collapse. As cleanup crews worked to clear the site, they realized the steel they were cutting had been the Towers' box columns (Figure 3)—hollow rectangular steel tubes that provided structural support for the Towers' distinctive façade.[13] The base of these torch-cut box columns that remain in bedrock[14] are now designated as historical remnants of September 11. They outline the Towers, allowing visitors to situate themselves in the underground space and to place themselves in relation to the buildings that once stood at this site.

The slurry wall, a key artifact of the site, tells an important story. A slurry wall is a civil engineering technique that constructs reinforced concrete walls in areas of soft earth close to open water to prevent the earth around a construction site from collapsing in on itself. After a vertical

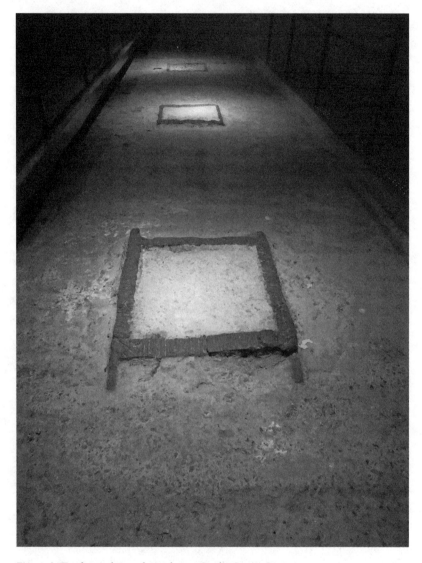

Figure 3. Torch-cut box column bases. Credit: Susan Opotow

wall is built, a building is constructed against it to hold up the wall and to keep pressure from the earth from pushing the slurry wall in. Before the World Trade Center could be built in 1966, a slurry wall had to be constructed to prevent water from seeping in and flooding the site. It was the first constructed in the United States.

Miraculously, when the Towers collapsed on 9/11, the slurry wall remained intact.[15] Had it been breached, damage to the site and the surrounding area would have been catastrophic. Architect Daniel Libeskind, master planner of the World Trade Center site, noted the symbolic significance of the slurry wall's remarkable integrity after the attacks: It had stood its ground when everything around it was collapsing. The slurry wall thus became a symbol of endurance.

The slurry wall is an important artifact of 9/11, but as Mark Wagner explained, preserving it proved challenging. Before 9/11, when the Twin Towers stood, the slurry wall had vertical earthen walls on one side and lateral floor slabs on the other to provide stability. On September 13, 2001, two days after the attacks, the wall remained intact, but engineers became concerned about its stability and, therefore, the stability of the site as a whole. With the towers gone, there was no structural element to hold up the slurry wall. This was not only a concern about preserving an historical artifact. Had the wall collapsed, a substantial part of Lower Manhattan, including the PATH tubes, the subways, and the West Side Highway could have been inundated by the Hudson River. However, debris from the buildings' collapse provided enough lateral bracing to hold up the wall initially. But as debris was removed, the potential for the slurry wall's collapse increased.

As Mark Wagner explained, rock anchors had been used to stabilize and brace the wall in its original construction in the 1960s, with the understanding that after construction of the World Trade Center, structural floor slabs would provide lateral bracing for the wall. Therefore the rock anchors were not meant to provide permanent stabilization and may have been detensioned after the construction was complete. After the collapse of the World Trade Center in 2001, the debris was so dense that it provided lateral bracing. As debris was being removed during the recovery and cleanup phase, new anchors were drilled through the wall and into the bedrock beyond, extending downward into the rock, sometimes more than 100 feet.

This presented the architects with an urgent design challenge. The void was central to the design of the museum, but it would be difficult to stabilize the slurry wall without adding slabs that would close off open space. This was resolved through a compromise. To stabilize the slurry wall, the construction crew installed permanent rock anchors that can withstand corrosion. They also installed a lean reinforcing structure on both sides of the wall to remove pressure on the wall. Visitors to the museum now see an exposed section of the original slurry wall, though it no longer does significant structural work (Figure 4).

The last column is an iconic artifact located at the center of Foundation Hall. It is the final steel beam cut down at the end of a nine-month recovery and cleanup process at the World Trade Center site on May 28, 2002,[16] and stood as a symbol of this effort at the May 30, 2002, ceremony at the World Trade Center site, with thousands in attendance.[17] For this occasion, it had been covered with poignant ephemera and inscriptions by recovery workers, first responders, volunteers, victims' relatives, and other people.

The last column had been identified as an important artifact for the museum early on: "There's no way we weren't going to take the last column," Mark Wagner said. The architects didn't know where the exhibit designers would place it, but they knew that adequate ceiling height was necessary and visitors needed to be able to view it from a distance as well as up close to appreciate its scale and significance (Figure 5). As visitors journey down the museum ramp now, they encounter the last column from multiple angles, first from above while standing on the ramp's balcony, next while descending to bedrock where they can visit it up close, and again after exiting the historic exhibition in the footprint of the North Tower.

Because the last column was covered with tributes, photos, and ephemera, preserving it was a challenge. It had been stored in Hangar 17 at the John F. Kennedy airport in Queens, New York along with other artifacts Mark Wagner had tagged from the pile, a challenging site for conservation because of humidity, salty sea air, and burning jet fuel.[18] Preserving the last column was a multistage and costly project.[19] Each object on all four sides of the column was measured and documented with photographs so it could be removed by art preservation conservator, Steven Weintraub, who made reproductions of the original items, which are now in protected storage. He obtained duplicate items (e.g., missing-persons posters, Mass cards, union decals) from family members and organizations, and he glued thin magnetic sheets to the back of duplicated and reproduced items so that they could be removed periodically to check on the last column's structural integrity.

Because the last column is situated near the slurry wall, which normally leaks a bit, and because of the large size of the void, tight controls

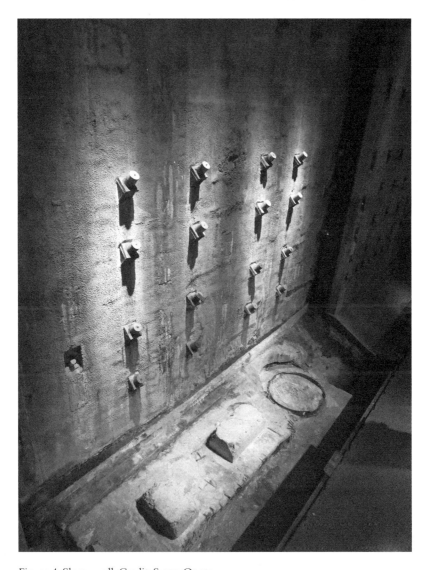

Figure 4. Slurry wall. Credit: Susan Opotow

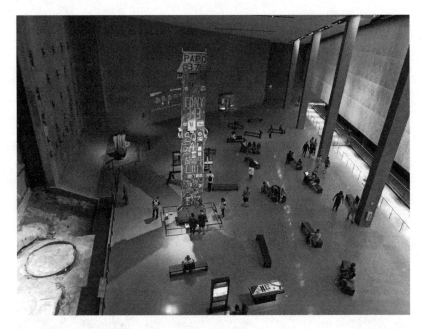

Figure 5. The "last column." Credit: Susan Opotow

of humidity and temperature are difficult to achieve, the last column's condition warrants close monitoring. Fifty-five percent relative humidity (plus or minus five points) would be ideal, but because the architects had no assurance that this could be consistently achieved, they designed a hatch that permits removal of the last column should adverse environmental conditions arise.

### Hurricane Sandy

Hurricane Sandy struck the Atlantic seaboard of the United States on October 29, 2012, at a time when construction of the museum was close to completion. All critical behind-the-scenes equipment (i.e., mechanical, electrical, and plumbing systems; disconnect switches; and sewer ejector pumps) was already in place at the lowest level of the museum. The museum's design included several ejector pits and pumps to remove water in case of flooding. To comply with code, an electrical disconnect switch had been installed next to these systems to shut them down quickly if needed. The night Hurricane Sandy bore down on New York City, the museum took in eight feet of water. Because the museum was an open construction site, water entered easily, and the intense storm surge overwhelmed the pumps. When rising water hit the disconnect switches, it burned everything out, flooding the museum, requiring extensive and costly repairs.[20]

*Building the Museum: People and Process*

In addition to design challenges of the September 11 Memorial Museum, the museum's development also included collaborations with many people and regulatory agencies.

The museum's developmental trajectory was unusual. Usually, architects meet with the museum director, curators, and historians who have already developed a narrative about what they want the museum to convey. But Davis Brody Bond received its commission to design the museum before it was formally created. They knew the site had a story that needed to be told, and they wanted people to experience the site on their own terms. They wanted a site with progressive disclosures that would open up to visitors as they descended the ramp into the void. And they wanted the big spaces to tell their own story and exhibitions situated in the footprints to offer an appropriate density of experience.

When museum director Alice Greenwald was hired in 2006, the architects had already completed design development. They realized they might need to revisit their plans after museum staff and the exhibit designer were hired, but that did not happen. Greenwald's goals were consistent with those of the architects. She wanted the museum to tell the story of what happened, attentive to the poignancy of the narrative, objects connected with it, and the site.[21]

There were, however, many occasions for disagreement and negotiation among the many stakeholders connected with World Trade Center site. As Mark Wagner described, differing perspectives on how the site should be developed could pit economic, administrative, practical, and emotional perspectives against each other. There were, for example, criticisms about the decision to build a memorial museum underground, and there were questions about whether the museum was being built too soon after 9/11.

Siting an historical museum at the World Trade Center site, he explained, required an historic preservation review mandated by Section 106 of the National Historic Preservation Act (NHPA) of 1966,[22] a process that takes into account the effects of construction or site modifications on historic properties. Once a site is approved as historically significant, all historical attributes named in the Memo of Understanding must be publicly accessible and preserved in perpetuity. For the September 11 Memorial Museum, the Section 106 Memo of Understanding listed footprints of the towers, the steel box beams, and, because of their significance in the preservation process, the anchor caps visible on the exposed original slurry wall.[23] Thus, even if the museum had been built on the plaza, as some stakeholders wanted, the designers still had a legal responsibility to provide public access to the lowest level because of its designation as a site of historical significance.

The Section 106 process also mandates that consulting parties be kept informed of design decisions. *Consulting parties* are people with any kind of vested interest in the work done on site. They may send a representative to meetings with the architects, and they can hire their own architects and consultants to review project details. Consulting parties for September 11 Memorial Museum included family members, local businesses, firefighters, police, and other kinds of groups, some small and others quite large. The architects presented periodic updates on the museum to 120 registered consulting parties. Though the consultative nature of this process could challenge design and construction decisions, over time, Mark Wagner said, the architects and consulting parties worked together to resolve pragmatic and emotional issues that emerged.

Reflecting back on his work at the World Trade Center site, Mark Wagner observed the importance of people, particularly the community that coalesced after September 11. He said,

> I am often asked what is the most important artifact to me personally. What is the one that resonates most for you? It was never an artifact. For me, it was about being on the site as part of this community; Red Cross workers offered hot meals after a long day or to wash my boots. And it was just a sense of community that we were all there together in a horrible place to be.

Throughout their work on the museum's design, the architects were attentive to people of the future and designed the museum as a site that could inspire learning, questioning, and contemplation for visitors from New York City or afar as well as for people who know a lot or a little about 9/11. Mark Wagner observed that many visitors, particularly those from elementary, middle, and high school, come to the museum without their own memories of 9/11. They learn about the significance of September 11, 2001, for the first time within a museum that conveys the traumatic history of destruction for people and the site itself.

## Linked Histories: People and Objects

Drawing on Mark Wagner's description of the museum's design and development, we discuss how the past and present, persons and objects, and history and memory are represented and intermingle in the September 11 Memorial Museum.

Pierre Nora has argued that history becomes necessary when people become conscious of the pastness of the past and need the aid of artifacts and documents to recall it.[24] Therefore sites of memory, such as museums, are created when familiar settings change or disappear to offer a space where memories and representations of the past can reside.[25] From this perspective, the September 11 Memorial Museum enables the shift from autobiographical to collective memories that Nora describes.[26] Paul Williams situates these functions as those of a memorial *museum,* "a specific kind of museum dedicated to a historic event commemorating mass suffering of some kind."[27] The September 11 Memorial Museum, located at the site of trauma, is now an important cultural site that historicizes and commemorates the attack on the Towers and the human fatalities and suffering that ensued.

Donald Winnicott has described a *holding environment* as a place of safety and trust.[28] Drawing on his construct, we see the museum's Foundation Hall as a holding environment for visitors within this memorial museum. Foundation Hall, with its vast size and soaring height, is the largest open space in the museum and an exhibition in its own right. It feels, as Mark Wagner described, like "walking into a cathedral with lighting that quiets you down; it does something to you emotionally." As an exhibition, it is spare, with only a few objects that survived in spite of a catastrophic past. Visitors cluster around the last column and other artifacts, listen at audio stations, but many simply sit in this space with subdued lighting, neutral colors, muted aluminum cladding that, together, evoke an atmosphere of reverence and sorrow. Loss is embodied in structural elements that originally had a mundane function but are now historic relics that invite scrutiny. The architects produced a space with an ethereal authenticity, consistent with the four design principles that guided Davis Brody Bond's work: memory, authenticity, scale, and emotion.[29]

Each artifact in Foundation Hall has its own story about the past. As the Twin Towers were transformed from building site in the 1960s to a site of commerce until 2001 to a ruin, a cleanup site, a rebuilding site, and then a museum, these objects were transformed as well. Their presence attests to that past, conveying the material and emotional history of the site.

Displayed as revered relics, they have historical, emotional, and symbolic significance. Each testifies to its past in this larger, intact and peopled site.

The idea that objects have permanence as they shift in meaning was observed by social psychologist Kurt Lewin in 1922. He proposed *genidentity* as a construct describing the genesis of an object from one moment to another. What we understand as an object, he explained, consists of multiple phases of the object at various times.[30] Genidentity names what visitors see at the museum: Objects that have been transformed since they were new. Visitors imaginatively interpret these physical transformations. The last column, for example, is one of many steel columns placed at the base of the World Trade Center's South Tower in the 1960s. Later it was covered with markings, pictures, and tributes by workers for the closing of the recovery operations in May 2002, and it now stands in a place of honor as a sentinel, symbol, and iconic object.

Kurt Lewin has also described social behavior and understanding occurring within what he called our *life space*, which results from an interaction between people and environment.[31] Mark Wagner had described the experience of this interaction when he descended the site access ramp at the World Trade Center during the cleanup period. He said, "It was an honor to go down that ramp every day, as hard as it was. I felt the emotional punch from my chest every time I did it, but I was glad to and felt I had to do it." The emotionally intense experience he describes connects his feeling to the thoughts of others as well as the specifics of the site. The subsequent design of the September 11 Memorial Museum visitor ramp also echoes attention to people and site, as Davis Brody Bond describes:[32]

> We chose as the space's main narrative element a gently descending procession (dubbed "the Ribbon") that guides visitors from the plaza to the bedrock level where the cut columns of the World Trade Center towers are revealed. The "ribbon" evokes the ramp used to remove debris from the site in the aftermath of the attacks. It also offers multiple views of the slurry wall, the original retaining wall that was built to withstand the lateral forces of landfill and river, and which survived the collapse of the towers. At the end of the ribbon, the descent continues down along the Vesey Street Stair ("Survivors' Stairs"), which were used by hundreds to escape to safety on 9/11. It ultimately leads to two exhibition spaces and Foundation Hall, the Museum's culminating space whose sheer scale conveys a sense of the enormity of the site and reinforces awareness of the absence of what once was there.

Their description evokes people from the past and present, including (in reverse chronological order): visitors, site workers after the Towers' collapse, survivors of 9/11 attack, and, by implication, the many people—office workers, rescue workers, and others—who did not survive.

Lewin's work grows out of Gestalt psychology, an innovative school of psychology that developed in Germany before World War II to research people's experience, perceptions, and the relations of parts to a whole.[33] A well-known Gestalt principle is that the whole is something other than the sum of its parts.[34] This principle applies at any scale: the whole of New York City is different than its many parts; the World Trade Center Site today is a civic entity that is different than its many buildings and functions; and the September 11 Memorial Museum has many parts, but they are not the same as the museum as a whole. Each element makes a distinctive contribution to the museum, and the interconnections among them yield a site with historical, perceptual, affective complexity.

Akin to this Gestalt principle is Manuel DeLanda's conceptualization of *assemblages,* which he defines as structural elements—spaces, objects, people, and technologies—that perform material as well as expressive roles.[35] DeLanda's work suggests that the September 11 Memorial can be understood as an *assemblage,* where each artifact (itself an assemblage) has material and affective meaning. Mark Wagner illustrated this idea when he described his role in developing the museum and the narrative importance of archival objects:

> At least fifteen of the large artifacts [from the pile of debris at the Twin Towers site] found their way into the museum, and that was one of the reasons why I was brought on: I understand the objects; I understood the story that they were going to tell, and I understood what it would take to move them all into the museum.

His observation succinctly conveys the mutually constitutive functions of material and expressive elements in the museum. Understanding the museum itself as an assemblage acknowledges how it simultaneously integrates people-environment, part-whole, and past-present relationships.

Similar to Gestalt psychology and assemblages, Patrizia Violi's work focused on the active role of the visitor in creating meaning in museums. She emphasizes the *indexical* character of material in sites of trauma.[36] Indexical objects are those whose meaning is dependent on context, and this context includes the museum history and setting as well as the visitors' own past. When visitors enter a museum where something terrible happened in the past, artifacts that embody this trauma—indexical objects—have the capacity to activate visitors' imagination to interpret what they see and understand, which also includes invisible and imagined traces of the past. As David Duindam has observed, because visitors anticipate seeing traces of the past at such sites, objects are indexical whether or not they are authentic to the time of trauma.[37] It is precisely such imaginative engagement, he and Violi propose, that fosters visitors' emotional engagement with the site and the past it represents. Mark Wagner also describes objects connected with September 11 as having autobiographical resonance:

> When we relate to an object, it brings us back to a time and a place in our lives or in somebody else's life so that we can then transpose our life into their life. Objects tell powerful stories. I can have a strong reaction to a fire truck and you might also have a strong reaction to it, but your cousin doesn't. We all connect with something differently.

Thus, everything in the September 11 Memorial Museum carries indexical meaning, whether or not they are artifacts of 2001. Elements of the museum, such as the ramp and rock anchors, both post–9/11, are nevertheless suffused with historical and emotional resonance.

When visitors give their attention to and engage with material evidence of the past—both site and objects—they position themselves as witnesses at a site of deadly violence where they can feel helpless because these events occurred in the past. Just as after the 9/11 attacks, when it was too late to help those who died,[38] it is also too late for visitors to take reparative action now. Yet, as Louise Purbrick describes, such visits are a "type of pilgrimage to a sacred landscape, which is completed within the museum."[39] By engaging with objects, the site, and its history at the September 11 Memorial Museum, a visitor, a bystander to past injustice, can develop a personal and empathic connection with a shocking, tragic past when seemingly inviolable buildings became dust and thousands perished at this site.

These theories that we bring to bear on the design, objects, and visitor experience at the September 11 Memorial Museum concern the psychological relevance of the environment, including objects, to human experience, emotions, and perception. Harold Searles articulated this in his psychoanalytic scholarship emphasizing the fundamental connection between people and the nonhuman environment as "one of the transcendentally important facts of human living."[40] In museums, but particularly in memorial museums that are sites of trauma, this connection takes on intensified meaning for objects seen as relics of that trauma. Thus, memorial museums work with design, narratives, and artifacts to support visitors' capacity to learn about and emphatically engage with a painful past.

## Conclusion

Combining history, design, culture, educational, commemorative, and touristic functions, memorial museums convey information as well as orient visitors to the meaning of significant events. Memorial museums began emerging in the late 1980s and have become increasingly prevalent since 2005.[41] However, as Paul Williams describes, memorial and museum functions are somewhat incompatible.[42] A memorial is designed to evoke reverent remembrance, while a museum is designed to provoke critical interpretation. Both these functions are evident at the September 11 Memorial Museum as artifacts displayed are simultaneously sacred because they survived to represent a violent past, while they are also instructional as they offer insight into that past.

Memorial museums have changed in style and approach over the past century. After World War I, they had a restrained aesthetic that dealt with death through allegory, avoiding ugly or shocking images. Memorial museums in Europe after World War II were largely way stations along pilgrimages to sites of battle.[43] Holocaust museums, which began emerging in the 1980s, have increasingly become features of many World War II museums.

The September 11 Memorial Museum, now a prominent cultural site in New York City, may continue to evolve over time. In most museums, permanent exhibitions are renovated periodically as aesthetics and technologies change; ensuing generations will form a different relationship to the past than people in the present; and even museum buildings change in response to emerging needs for space or as the result of damage. As a cultural genre, memorial museums may also change to align with emerging sensibilities about representations of violence and death, as happened in the last century. Thus, the September 11 Memorial Museum itself can be understood in light of genidentity, Kurt Lewin's 1922 observation we have described: that objects have permanence while they also shift in meaning.[44]

Not only will the September 11 Memorial Museum, a fresh and important cultural institution, increasingly represent the historical, physical, and emotional past of September 11 for future generations, but it is also our hope that as contemporary memories become history, the chapters in this book will speak to future generations as well.

## Notes

The authors appreciate the assistance of Tom Hennes and Neil Clarke, and we especially thank Mark Wagner for his advice and contributions to this chapter.

1. The History Channel, "World Trade Center." Available at https://goo.gl/raqJk9.

2. The World Trade Center (WTC) Health Program: Program Statistics. Available at https://goo.gl/jf7e95. See also "Health Impacts of 9/11" in this book.

3. September 11 Memorial Museum Mission statement. Available at https://goo.gl/7zUcCN.

4. Images and a cross-sectional sketch of the museum are available at https://goo.gl/6zqHED.

5. Video of the Memorial Exhibition is available at https://goo.gl/3EfzG2.

6. Layman joined the project in 2010. Information on the historical exhibition is available at: https://goo.gl/xRQP2o. Information on the architects involved in building the museum is available at https://goo.gl/Hrzyc2.

7. Michael Shulan served as the museum's creative director at the time that the Memorial and historical exhibitions were being developed.

8. See Sturken, 2004, 2015, 2016. A timeline of the World Trade Center is available at https://goo.gl/rTB6Tj.

9. Opotow 2011a, 2011b, 2015.

10. Cleanup and recovery video: https://goo.gl/Vt1CFe.

11. Eric Lipton and James Glanz, "A Nation Challenged: Relics; From the Rubble, Artifacts of Anguish," *New York Times*, January 27, 2002.

12. See Sagalyn, 2016, 356–357, on contentious infrastructure issues (i.e., cost, politics) at Ground Zero.

13. David W. Dunlap, "Twin Towers Column Stubs, Once Amputated, Are Now Being Protected," *New York Times*, March 22, 2006.

14. Mark Wagner: "The term 'bedrock' is used loosely. The cut box columns were embedded in the concrete slab on grade. The slab sat on a bed of gravel, the gravel on earth/dirt/ grade and the earth on the actual rock . . . bedrock. The columns were welded to steel base plates, which were bolted to a concrete footing called a grade beam, the grade beam sat on bedrock. The bedrock was not visible until the design called for excavation to reveal it."

15. David W. Dunlap, "Looking to a Wall That Limited the Devastation at the World Trade Center," *New York Times*, September 11, 2013.

16. Sturken, 2015.

17. Images and text on the last column are available at https://goo.gl/W3XojT. A video is at https://goo.gl/d7nhuP.

18. David W. Dunlap, "Once Filled With Symbols of Hope and Despair, a 9/11 Repository Is Set to Close," *New York Times,* May 18, 2016.

19. David W. Dunlap, "Halting Rust From Devouring What 9/11 Couldn't: Curators Battle Elements to Preserve Pieces of a Terrible History," *New York Times,* April 3, 2004.

20. David W. Dunlap, "Floodwater Pours Into 9/11 Museum, Hampering Further Work on the Site," *New York Times,* November 2, 2012; Alice M. Greenwald, "Our Beacon of Hope," *9/11 Memorial & Museum Blog,* December 7, 2012, available at https://goo.gl/FxiW46.

21. Greenwald, 2010, 2016.

22. For the text of the National Historic Preservation Act of 1966 (NHPA), see https://goo.gl/k3xGE8. The Advisory Council on Historic Preservation is described at https://goo.gl/FfUcXe.

23. Mark Wagner: "Only the anchor caps that are visible on the surface of the exposed original slurry wall are protected under the 106 Memo of Understanding. These were not permanent anchors. These were the temporary anchors installed post 9/11 to stabilize the wall during the debris removal process and until a permanent structural solution could be designed."

24. Nora, 1996; Ho Tai, 2001.

25. Risnicoff de Gorgas, 2001.

26. Halbwachs, 1992.

27. Williams, 2007, 8.

28. Winnicott, 1972.

29. Karissa Rosenfield, "9/11 Memorial Museum/Davis Brody Bond," *Arch-Daily,* March 21, 2014: https://goo.gl/mULRsn.

30. Lewin, 1922; Smith and Mulligan, 1982.

31. Deutsch, 1954; Lewin, 1935.

32. See https://goo.gl/BUeq3c.

33. Ash, 1995.

34. Often mistranslated as "The whole is more than the sum of its parts." Gestalt psychologist Kurt Koffka (1935, 176) described summing as a meaningless procedure; instead, whole-part relationships are what is meaningful.

35. DeLanda, 2006; Price-Robertson and Duff, 2016.

36. Violi, 2012.

37. Duindam, 2016.

38. James Glanz and Eric Lipton, "A Nation Challenged: The Site; The Excavation: Planning, Precision and Pain," *New York Times,* September 27, 2001.

39. Purbrick, 2011, 171.

40. Searles, 1960, 6.

41. Williams, 2007.

42. Ibid.

43. Winter, 2012.

44. Lewin, 1922; Smith and Mulligan, 1982.

## References

Aronson, Jay D. *Who Owns the Dead? The Science and Politics of Death at Ground Zero.* Cambridge, MA: Harvard University Press, 2016.

Ash, Mitchell G. *Gestalt Psychology in German Culture, 1890–1967: Holism and the Quest for Objectivity.* New York: Cambridge University Press, 1995.

DeLanda, Manuel. *A New Philosophy of Society: Assemblage Theory and Social Complexity.* London: Continuum, 2006.

Deutsch, Morton. "Field Theory in Social Psychology." *Handbook of Social Psychology* 1 (1954): 181–222.

Duindam, David, "Sign of the Shoah: The Hollandsche Schouwburg as a Site of Memory." Doctoral dissertation, University of Amsterdam, 2016.

Greenwald, Alice M. "'Passion on All Sides': Lessons for Planning the National September 11 Memorial Museum." *Curator: The Museum Journal* 53, no. 1 (2010): 117–125.

Greenwald, Alice M., ed. *No Day Shall Erase You: The Story of 9/11 as Told at the National September 11 Memorial Museum.* New York: 9/11 Memorial/Skira Rizzoli, 2016.

Halbwachs, Maurice. *On Collective Memory.* University of Chicago Press, 1992.

Ho Tai, Hue-Tam. "Remembered Realms: Pierre Nora and French National Memory." *American Historical Review* 106, no. 3 (2001): 906–922.

Koffka, Kurt. *Principles of Gestalt Psychology.* New York: Harcourt, Brace, 1935.

Lewin, Kurt. *Der Begriff der Genese in Physik, Biologie und Entwicklungsgeschichte* (The Concept of Genesis in Physics, Biology, and the History of Development). Berlin: Springer, 1922.

———. *A Dynamic Theory of Personality: Selected Papers.* New York: McGraw-Hill, 1935.

Nora, Pierre. *Realms of Memory: The Construction of the French Past.* New York: Columbia University Press, 1996.

Opotow, Susan. "How This Was Possible: Interpreting the Holocaust." *Journal of Social Issues* 67, no. 1 (2011a): 205–224.

———. "Absence and Presence: Interpreting Moral Exclusion in the Jewish Museum Berlin." In *Justice and Conflicts: Theoretical and Empirical Contributions,* edited by Elisabeth Kals and Jürgen Maes, 53–74. Dordrecht: Springer, 2011b.

———. "Historicizing Injustice: The Museum of Memory and Human Rights, Santiago, Chile." *Journal of Social Issues,* 71, no. 2 (2015): 229–243.

Price-Robertson, Rhys, and Cameron Duff. "Realism, Materialism, and the Assemblage: Thinking Psychologically with Manuel DeLanda." *Theory & Psychology* 26, no. 1 (2016): 58–76.

Purbrick, Louise. "Museums and the Embodiment of Human Rights." *Museum and Society* 9, no. 3 (2011): 166–189.

Risnicoff de Gorgas, Mónica. "Reality as Illusion: The Historic Houses That Become Museums." *Museum International* 53, no. 2 (2001): 10–15.

Sagalyn, Lynne B. *Power at Ground Zero: Politics, Money, and the Remaking of Lower Manhattan.* New York: Oxford University Press, 2016.

Smith, Barry, and Mulligan, Kevin (1982) Pieces of a Theory, §6. In *Parts and Moments: Studies in Logic and Formal Ontology,* edited by B. Smith, 15–110. Munich: Philosophia.

Sturken, Marita. "The Aesthetics of Absence: Rebuilding Ground Zero." *American Ethnologist* 31, no. 3 (2004): 311–325.

———. "The 9/11 Memorial Museum and the Remaking of Ground Zero." *American Quarterly* 67, no. 2 (2015): 471–90.

———. "The Objects That Lived: The 9/11 Museum and Material Transformation." *Memory Studies* 9, no. 1 (2016): 13–26.

Violi, Patrizia. "Trauma Site Museums and Politics of Memory: Tuol Sleng, Villa Grimaldi and the Bologna Ustica Museum." *Theory, Culture & Society* 29, no. 1 (2012): 36–75.

Williams, Paul Harvey. *Memorial Museums: The Global Rush to Commemorate Atrocities*. New York: Berg, 2007.

Winnicott, Donald W. *Holding and Interpretation: Fragment of an Analysis*. New York: Grove Press, 1972.

Winter, Jay. "Museums and the Representation of War." *Museum and Society* 10, no. 3 (2012): 150–163.

# Acknowledgments

The origins of this book lie in the first days after September 11, 2001, when it was unclear what would happen next. To understand the sequelae of this terrifying attack of the World Trade Center, I began studying the news, clipping *New York Times* articles on New York City that detailed issues emerging in 9/11's wake. I was a faculty member in the Graduate Program in Dispute Resolution at the University of Massachusetts Boston at that time, and I greatly appreciated discussing and analyzing these articles with the assistance of graduate students Jerry Fletcher, Sarah Gyorog, Vicki Myers, and Sarah Woodside and statistician Jie Chen.

When I joined the City University of New York's Sociology Department of John Jay College of Criminal Justice and PhD Program in Social/Personality Psychology of The Graduate Center, doctoral students Zachary Shemtob (coeditor of this book), Patrick Sweeney, Kate Sheese, and Lorraine Phillips joined me to examine the changes that 9/11 wrought in New York over time. I am grateful for their assistance.

I am most appreciative of four grants I received to advance this project: the American Psychological Foundation's Raymond A. and Rosalee G. Weiss Innovative Research and Program Grant for "After 9/11: Psychological Conflict, Challenge, and Change in New York City, 2001–2006" (2008); the Office for the Advancement of Research at John Jay College of Criminal Justice grant for "The Post–9/11 Period in New York City" (2008–2009); the PSC-CUNY Award jointly funded by the Professional Staff Congress and The City University of New York for "Developing the 9/11 Memorial Museum: Conflicts and Challenges" (2010); and the

Book Publication Funding Award from the Office for the Advancement of Research at John Jay College of Criminal Justice, City University of New York (2015).

A direct precursor for this book was a half-day conference, "9/11 Plus Ten: New York City in the Aftermath of September 11," that Zachary Shemtob and I organized to commemorate the tenth anniversary of the 2001 attacks. Held at The Graduate Center, City University of New York, it was open to the public. Its panels on Rebuilding Ground Zero, Muslim Citizens in the Wounded City, and 9/11's Aftermath: Health, Safety, and Change were well received. We thank Katherine Carl of the Center for the Humanities for collaborating with us in organizing this event and Graduate Center President Chase Robinson for being part of it. We also thank panelists Norman Groner, Daniel Libeskind, and Michael Arad, outstanding speakers at the conference, who wrote chapters for this book.

All the book's authors are impressive and have been generous with their time and expertise. We are grateful for their incisive chapters and moved by their conviction that an analysis of 9/11's aftermath is an important endeavor.

Coeditor and coauthor Zachary Shemtob has been a wonderful collaborator because of his gift for writing, his editorial acumen, and his unflagging commitment to this project.

We appreciate the assistance of many people who have contributed to this book in various ways. They include Michelle Fine, Jennifer Chemielewski, Dan Perlman, Chris Kelaher, Michael Sovkin, Dan Stageman, Sandra Rutherford, Amanda de Beaufort, Micki Siegel, Kimberly Flynn, Ramzi Kassem, Jonathan Kingley, Eunjoo Byeon, Neil Clarke, Mark Wagner, Tom Hennes, and Richard Clark.

Finally, we thank the terrific editorial staff at Fordham University Press: Will Cerbone, Ann-Christine Racette, Eric Newman, and Gregory McNamee. It's been a pleasure to work with them.

*—Susan Opotow*

In addition to acknowledging my appreciation to all of the folks mentioned above, I would be remiss in not thanking my fantastic collaborator and coeditor, Susan, for getting me involved in the early stages of what eventually became this project.

*—Zachary Baron Shemtob*

# Contributors

**Michael Arad,** B.A., M.Arch., AIA, is best known for his design for the National September 11 Memorial at the World Trade Center site, titled "Reflecting Absence," which was selected by the Lower Manhattan Development Corporation from among more than 5,000 entries submitted in an international competition held in 2003. Arad joined the New York firm of Handel Architects as a partner in April 2004, where he worked on realizing the Memorial design as a member of the firm. A native of Israel, Arad was raised there, the United Kingdom, the United States, and Mexico. He came to the United States and earned his B.A. from Dartmouth College in 1994 and M.Arch. from the Georgia Institute of Technology in 1999. In 2006, he was one of six recipients of the Young Architects Award of the American Institute of Architects. In 2012, he was awarded the AIA Presidential Citation for his work on the National September 11 Memorial.

**Michael Crane,** M.D., M.P.H., is medical director of the Selikoff Centers for Occupational Health, the Mount Sinai World Trade Center Health Program Clinical Center of Excellence, and associate professor of the Department of Environmental Medicine and Public Health at the Icahn School of Medicine at Mount Sinai. He is an expert on the physical and mental health consequences of large-scale disasters experienced by rescue and recovery workers including responders who worked at the World Trade Center disaster site following the attacks of September 11, 2001. An advocate of worker safety and health, Dr. Crane has conducted extensive research on the health effects of exposures to workplace hazards and environmental toxins, as well as on prevention and control strategies to protect worker health.

**Brian R. Davis,** M.A., M.Phil., is a doctoral candidate in Social/Personality Psychology at The Graduate Center, City University of New York (CUNY), and a Fulbright Dissertation Research Fellow to Osaka Prefecture University, Japan (2016–17). He currently serves as graduate student board member at the LGBT Social Science & Public Policy Center at Roosevelt House, Hunter College (CUNY), as well as liaison to Japan for the International Psychology Network for LGBTI Issues (IPsyNet). His mixed qualitative and quantitative methods research focuses on sexual identity development, adolescent sexuality, minority stress, and policy applications. His dissertation project focuses on exploring the culturally contingent beliefs about male sexuality in the United States and Japan.

**Ariel Durosky,** B.A., is the research coordinator of the Trauma and PTSD program at the New York State Psychiatric Institute at Columbia University Medical Center. She earned a B.A. in psychology from Emmanuel College and previously conducted research related to sex differences in leadership styles.

**Kimberly Flynn,** B.A., is the cofounder and director of 9/11 Environmental Action, a key advocacy organization that formed in 2002 as a community-based coalition to call attention to the environmental health risks of the WTC disaster and to advocate for a proper cleanup. The organization aims to ensure that residents, workers and students (a.k.a. "survivors") who were affected physically or emotionally by the WTC disaster get the health care they need and deserve. For more than five years, she has been the chair of the Survivors Steering Committee, an advisory body whose mission is to provide input from the affected community to the World Trade Center Health Program's Survivor Program. She has served on numerous 9/11 health-related committees, including the WTC Scientific/Technical Advisory Committee, where she participated in the deliberation resulting in a recommendation that the WTCHP add more than 50 cancers to the list of WTC conditions.

**Norman Groner,** Ph.D., is an emeritus professor at John Jay College of Criminal Justice, CUNY, affiliated with the Department of Security, Fire and Emergency Management. He has taught a wide variety of courses related to security, emergency management, fire safety, and research methods.

He earned his doctorate in research psychology from the University of Washington. His scholarly writing and research concerns the cognitive and organizational factors related to fire safety, security, and emergency planning. Groner has investigated human behavior during fires, conducted studies of organizational responses during disasters, analyzed the feasibility of using building refuge areas and fire-safe elevators, worked on various task forces and code writing committees, and advised the National Institute of Standards and Technology on data collection and analysis for its investigation of the evacuations of the World Trade Center on September 11, 2001.

**Liat Helpman,** Ph.D., is a postdoctoral fellow. She is a member of the Trauma and PTSD program at the New York State Psychiatric Institute at Columbia University Medical Center. She is also a part of the Columbia Global Mental Health team, working to improve access to evidence-based interventions among internally displaced women in Colombia. Dr. Helpman is investigating biomarkers of stress and translating research into practical applications. She has expertise in clinical practice with adults and children with PTSD and other clinical problems.

**Anne Hilburn,** M.A., is a research assistant with the Trauma and PTSD Program at the New York State Psychiatric Institute at Columbia University Medical Center.

**Charles Jennings,** Ph.D., FIFireE, CFO, is a public safety academic and researcher, and practitioner. He is inaugural director of the Christian Regenhard Center for Emergency Response Studies (RaCERS) at John Jay College of Criminal Justice, where he is also an associate professor in the Department of Security, Fire, and Emergency Management. He has an extensive background as a public safety practitioner and researcher.

**Daniel Libeskind,** B.Arch., M.A., BDA, FAIA, is an international figure in architecture and urban design. He is renowned for his ability to evoke cultural memory in buildings and is informed by a deep commitment to music, philosophy, and literature. Libeskind aims to create architecture that is resonant, original, and sustainable. Born in Lódz, Poland, in 1946, Mr. Libeskind immigrated to the United States as a teenager. He established his architectural studio in Berlin, Germany, in 1989 after winning the competition to build the Jewish Museum there. In February 2003, when Libeskind was selected as the master planner for the World Trade Center redevelopment, he moved from Berlin to New York City. His

Studio Libeskind has completed buildings that range from museums and concert halls to convention centers, university buildings, hotels, shopping centers and residential towers. As principal design architect for Studio Libeskind, he speaks widely on the art of architecture in universities and at professional summits. His architecture and ideas have been the subject of many articles and exhibitions, influencing the field of architecture and the development of cities and culture. Libeskind lives in New York with his wife and business partner, Nina Libeskind.

**Ari Lowell,** Ph.D., is associate director of the Columbia Veterans Research Center, a part of the Trauma and PTSD Program at the New York State Psychiatric Institute at Columbia University Medical Center. He has a background in treating PTSD, depression, anxiety, and traumatic brain injury. He completed his clinical internship at the VA NJ Health Care System, where he served veterans suffering from the effects of combat-related trauma, military sexual trauma, and other difficulties. Lowell is experienced in both individual and group psychotherapy. He is a veteran of the Israel Defense Forces.

**Roberto Lucchini,** M.D., has since 2012 been director of the Division of Occupational Medicine, professor of medicine, director of the World Trade Center, Data Center, and director of NIOSH Education and Research Center for New York and New Jersey. He is also associate professor at the University of Brescia, Italy, Division of Occupational Medicine. He is committed to sharing his knowledge internationally and promoting the center's research on the assessment of health outcomes among the World Trade Center responders who were exposed to a variety of chemical hazards and psychological trauma at Ground Zero.

**Guillermina Mejia,** M.P.H., was the director of the Safety and Health Department of District Council 37, AFSCME and an experienced Occupational Safety and Health Specialist. District Council 37 is a labor organization that represents city, state, and cultural workers. Many of its members performed a variety of tasks at Ground Zero, the surrounding areas, and the landfill. Since 9/11, Ms. Mejia has worked on getting New York City to protect District Council 37's members from the safety and health hazards that resulted from 9/11, and she has advocated for medical support for those injured and exposed to toxic environments. Ms. Mejia was a member of the WTC HP Responder Steering Committee and served on the WTC Scientific and Technical Advisory Committee.

**Hirofumi Minami**, Ph.D., is professor of environmental psychology in the Department of Urban Design and Disaster Management at the Faculty of Human-Environment Studies of Kyushu University, Japan. He specializes in developmental and environmental psychology, urban design, and cultural psychology. His research topics include childhood memories of significant places, urban renewal and the elderly, cultural assumptions underlying environmental concepts, social ecological studies of urban life in Asian cities, ethnographic and field research methods, and Psychoanalysis of Cities. He cofounded the Japanese Society of Qualitative Psychology, chaired the Man-Environment Research Association, and was dean of the Faculty of Education of Kyushu University.

**Jacqueline Moline**, M.D., M.Sc., is an occupational medicine specialist and has published widely on the physical and mental health effects of World Trade Center exposure observed within the Mount Sinai Clinical Program. Her involvement in medical monitoring and treatment of WTC responders began in 2002, when she became the Medical Core Director of the WTC Worker and Volunteer Medical Screening Program. She joined North Shore in April 2010 as vice president of population health and was the founding chair of population health for the new Hofstra School of Medicine. Dr. Moline works with the health system leadership to develop initiatives aimed at promoting and engaging health and wellness for North Shore-LIJ's workforce as well as community at large. She is also developing a population health and epidemiology research program. Dr. Moline's research in the past has focused on the health effects of lead exposure.

**Yuval Neria**, Ph.D., is professor of medical psychology at the Departments of Psychiatry and Epidemiology at Columbia University Medical Center, and Director of Trauma and PTSD at the New York State Psychiatric Institute. His research ranges from studying the mental health consequences of high impact trauma including combat, captivity, terrorism and disasters, examination of determinants of resilience and effective functioning, to translational research aiming to identify underlying neural and behavioral mechanisms of trauma related psychopathology and development of neuroscience-informed treatments.

**Cristina Onea**, M.A., is a Ph.D. student in the Critical Social and Personality Psychology program at the Graduate Center at the City University of New York. She draws upon her background as a Romanian immigrant for inspiration in her research. Cristina is currently studying surveillance

as well as transgenerational trauma as a result of mass human rights viola-
tions. She is interested in the effects of surveillance on social relationships,
trust, and the physical and mental well-being of the individual.

**Susan Opotow,** Ph.D., is a professor at City University of New York, where
she is a core faculty member of sociology at John Jay College and psychology at the Graduate Center. A social psychologist, her research examines
the psychology of justice, conflict, exclusion, and inclusion. She is a Fellow of the American Psychological Association, heads the Ph.D. Program
in Critical Social/Personality Psychology at the Graduate Center, and is
the 2018 Chair of the Board for the Advancement of Psychology in the
Public Interest of the American Psychological Association. She was editor
of *Peace and Conflict: Journal of Peace Psychology* (2010–2013) and president
of the Society for the Psychological Study of Social Issues (2008–2009).

**David Prezant,** M.D., is the Chief Medical Officer for the Fire Department of the City of New York FDNY), a special advisor to the Fire Commissioner on health policy, and codirector of the FDNY World Trade
Center Medical Monitoring Program. He is also professor of medicine at
the Albert Einstein College of Medicine. On 9/11, Dr. Prezant responded
to the World Trade Center and was present during the collapse and its
aftermath. Since that day, he has worked to initiate a multimillion-dollar
medical monitoring and treatment program for FDNY firefighters funded
by FDNY, the Centers for Disease Control and Prevention (CDC), and
the National Institute for Occupational Safety and Health (NIOSH). His
major research interest is in determining the mechanisms responsible for
accelerated decline in longitudinal pulmonary function and/or airway
hyperreactivity in firefighters after WTC exposure. Other interests are in
determining the mechanisms responsible for the increased incidence of
sarcoidosis in firefighters after WTC exposure.

**Karyna Pryiomka** is a doctoral candidate in the Critical Social/Personality
Psychology Ph.D. program and has earned the Interactive Technology and
Pedagogy Graduate Certificate at the Graduate Center, CUNY. Drawing
on the history of psychology and the philosophy of science, Karyna's research interests include the relationship between psychological assessments
and education policy, validity theory, and the qualitative/quantitative
divide in social science research. Her work on digital pedagogy has appeared in the *Journal of Interactive Technology and Pedagogy* (2017), and her
theoretical work has been published in *the Moscow State Herald* (2015). She

brings these interests and a blend of critical and digital pedagogies into her teaching of psychology and statistical methods courses at the City University of New York.

**Joan Reibman**, M.D., is the medical director of the World Trade Center Environmental Health Center and director of the New York University/ Bellevue Asthma Clinic, as well as professor in the Department of Medicine and Environmental Medicine at New York University. In 1991, she began the Bellevue Hospital Asthma program under a New York grant. She uses the research in both research centers to promote the study of airway disease and environmental interactions. Under Dr. Reibman's supervision, these labs were the first to study the environmental impact of the destruction of the World Trade Center towers on the respiratory health of the surrounding community.

**Diala Shamas** is a human rights attorney whose practice and writing focus on civil liberties, law enforcement accountability, and lawyering in support of communities impacted by policies pursued under the banner of national security. She is a staff attorney at the Center for Constitutional Rights in New York, and has taught at Stanford Law School and at CUNY School of Law.

**Zachary Baron Shemtob**, Ph.D., J.D., is a practicing lawyer and former assistant professor of criminology and criminal justice at Central Connecticut State University. He earned his J.D. from Georgetown University Law Center in 2015; his Ph.D. and M.Phil. in Criminal Justice from the Graduate Center of the City of New York in 2011; his M.A. from John Jay College of Criminal Justice in 2009; and his B.A. from Wesleyan University in 2006. He specializes and has written on theories of punishment, jurisprudence, and the death penalty.

**Micki Siegel de Hernández**, M.P.H., is the health and safety director for the Communications Workers of America (CWA), District 1. CWA represents an extremely diverse group of workers in both the public and private sectors, thousands of whom were responders, as well as survivors, of the 9/11 disaster. She became Chair of the WTC Health Program (WTCHP) Responder Steering Committee in February 2018 after serving as a labor representative on the RSC since its inception. She currently serves on the WTC Scientific and Technical Advisory Committee established under the Zadroga Act. She is also a labor representative on the

WTCHP Survivor Program Steering Committee, has served as a labor representative on the NYC DOHMH WTC Registry Labor Advisory Committee, was the labor liaison on the EPA WTC Expert Technical Review Panel, and was the labor co-chair of the WTC Community/ Labor Coalition.

**Patrick Sweeney**, M.A., M.Phil., is a doctoral candidate in Critical Social Psychology at the Graduate Center, CUNY; and a Digital Fellow at the GC Digital Scholarship lab. His research examines media, technology, social categories, and justice. You can find out more about his work at http://patricksweeney.info.

**Xi Zhu**, Ph.D., is a research scientist with the Trauma and PTSD program at the New York State Psychiatric Institute at Columbia University Medical Center. She has a background in imaging processing, machine learning, computational modeling, and big data analytics. Her current research focuses on utilizing resting state fMRI, structural MRI, diffusion tensor imaging (DTI), and task fMRI to identify brain biomarkers of PTSD. She is also interested in integrating large-scale datasets across many different types and using a machine learning/Artificial Intelligence approach to construct predictive network models and predict treatment outcome.

# Index

Page numbers in italics denote illustrations, and the letter *t* following a page number denotes a table. The following abbreviations are used in the index:

| | |
|---|---|
| *Memorial* | National September 11 Memorial |
| *Memorial and Museum* | National September 11 Memorial and Museum |
| *Memorial Museum* | National September 11 Memorial Museum |
| *NYC* | New York City |
| *NYPD* | New York Police Department |
| *PTSD* | posttraumatic stress disorder |
| *US* | United States |
| *WTC* | World Trade Center |

**ESE** SELECT TITLES FROM EMPIRE STATE EDITIONS

Andrew J. Sparberg, *From a Nickel to a Token: The Journey from Board of Transportation to MTA*

Daniel Campo, *The Accidental Playground: Brooklyn Waterfront Narratives of the Undesigned and Unplanned*

John Waldman, *Heartbeats in the Muck: The History, Sea Life, and Environment of New York Harbor, Revised Edition*

John Waldman (ed.), *Still the Same Hawk: Reflections on Nature and New York*

Gerard R. Wolfe, *The Synagogues of New York's Lower East Side: A Retrospective and Contemporary View, Second Edition*. Photographs by Jo Renée Fine and Norman Borden, Foreword by Joseph Berger

Joseph B. Raskin, *The Routes Not Taken: A Trip Through New York City's Unbuilt Subway System*

Phillip Deery, *Red Apple: Communism and McCarthyism in Cold War New York*

*North Brother Island: The Last Unknown Place in New York City*. Photographs by Christopher Payne, A History by Randall Mason, Essay by Robert Sullivan

Stephen Miller, *Walking New York: Reflections of American Writers from Walt Whitman to Teju Cole*

Tom Glynn, *Reading Publics: New York City's Public Libraries, 1754–1911*

Craig Saper, *The Amazing Adventures of Bob Brown: A Real-Life Zelig Who Wrote His Way Through the 20th Century*

R. Scott Hanson, *City of Gods: Religious Freedom, Immigration, and Pluralism in Flushing, Queens*. Foreword by Martin E. Marty

Mark Naison and Bob Gumbs, *Before the Fires: An Oral History of African American Life in the Bronx from the 1930s to the 1960s*

Robert Weldon Whalen, *Murder, Inc., and the Moral Life: Gangsters and Gangbusters in La Guardia's New York*

Joanne Witty and Henrik Krogius, *Brooklyn Bridge Park: A Dying Waterfront Transformed*

Sharon Egretta Sutton, *When Ivory Towers Were Black: A Story about Race in America's Cities and Universities*

Pamela Hanlon, *A Wordly Affair: New York, the United Nations, and the Story Behind Their Unlikely Bond*

Britt Haas, *Fighting Authoritarianism: American Youth Activism in the 1930s*

David J. Goodwin, *Left Bank of the Hudson: Jersey City and the Artists of 111 1st Street*. Foreword by DW Gibson

Nandini Bagchee, *Counter Institution: Activist Estates of the Lower East Side*

Carol Lamberg, *Neighborhood Success Stories: Creating and Sustaining Affordable Housing in New York*

Susan Celia Greenfield (ed.), *Sacred Shelter: Thirteen Journeys of Homelessness and Healing*

Elizabeth Macaulay Lewis and Matthew McGowan (eds.), *Classical New York: Discovering Greece and Rome in Gotham*

Andrew Feffer, *Bad Faith: Teachers, Liberalism, and the Origins of McCarthyism*

**For a complete list, visit www.empirestateeditions.com.**